2 x 4/05 v 7/05

Understanding
Headaches
and Migraines

D0972903

APR 2 3 2004

Understanding Illness and Health

Many health problems and worries are strongly influenced by our thoughts and feelings. These exciting new books, written by experts in the psychology of health, are essential reading for sufferers, their families and friends.

Each book presents objective, easily understood information and advice about what the problem is, the treatments available and, most importantly, how your state of mind can help or hinder the way you cope. You will discover how to have a positive, hopeful outlook, which will help you choose the most effective treatment for you and your particular lifestyle, with confidence.

The series is edited by JANE OGDEN, Reader in Health Psychology, Guy's, King's and St Thomas' School of Medicine, King's College London, UK.

Titles in the series

KAREN BALLARD Understanding Menopause

SIMON DARNLEY & BARBARA MILLAR Understanding Irritable Bowel Syndrome

LINDA PAPADOPOULOS & CARL WALKER Understanding Skin Problems

PENNY TITMAN Understanding Childhood Eczema

MARIE CLARK Understanding Diabetes

MARK FORSHAW Understanding Headaches and Migraines

Understanding Headaches and Migraines

MARK FORSHAW

SAN DIEGO PUBLIC LIBRARY
LA JOLLA BRANCH

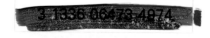

3 1336 06473 4874

John Wiley & Sons, Ltd

Copyright © 2004   John Wiley & Sons Ltd, The Atrium, Southern Gate, Chichester, West Sussex PO19 8SQ, England

Telephone (+44) 1243 779777

Email (for orders and customer service enquiries): cs-books@wiley.co.uk
Visit our Home Page on www.wileyeurope.com or www.wiley.com

All Rights Reserved. No part of this publication may be reproduced, stored in a retrieval system or transmitted in any form or by any means, electronic, mechanical, photocopying, recording, scanning or otherwise, except under the terms of the Copyright, Designs and Patents Act 1988 or under the terms of a licence issued by the Copyright Licensing Agency Ltd, 90 Tottenham Court Road, London W1T 4LP, UK, without the permission in writing of the Publisher. Requests to the Publisher should be addressed to the Permissions Department, John Wiley & Sons Ltd, The Atrium, Southern Gate, Chichester, West Sussex PO19 8SQ, England, or emailed to permreq@wiley.co.uk, or faxed to (+44) 1243 770620.

This publication is designed to provide accurate and authoritative information in regard to the subject matter covered. It is sold on the understanding that the Publisher is not engaged in rendering professional services. If professional advice or other expert assistance is required, the services of a competent professional should be sought.

Other Wiley Editorial Offices

John Wiley & Sons Inc., 111 River Street, Hoboken, NJ 07030, USA

Jossey-Bass, 989 Market Street, San Francisco, CA 94103-1741, USA

Wiley-VCH Verlag GmbH, Boschstr. 12, D-69469 Weinheim, Germany

John Wiley & Sons Australia Ltd, 33 Park Road, Milton, Queensland 4064, Australia

John Wiley & Sons (Asia) Pte Ltd, 2 Clementi Loop #02-01, Jin Xing Distripark, Singapore 129809

John Wiley & Sons Canada Ltd, 22 Worcester Road, Etobicoke, Ontario, Canada M9W 1L1

Wiley also publishes its books in a variety of electronic formats. Some content that appears in print may not be available in electronic books.

Library of Congress Cataloging-in-Publication Data

Forshaw, Mark.
  Understanding headaches and migraines / Mark Forshaw.
    p. cm. – (Understanding illness & health)
Includes bibliographical references and index.
  ISBN 0-470-84760-3 (Paper : alk. paper)
 1. Headache. 2. Migraine. 3. Consumer education. I. Title. II.
Series.
  RC392.F676 2004
  616.8′491–dc22

                                 2003018655

British Library Cataloguing in Publication Data

A catalogue record for this book is available from the British Library

ISBN 0-470-84760-3

Typeset in 10/13.5pt Photina by Laserwords Private Limited, Chennai, India
Printed and bound in Great Britain by TJ International, Padstow, Cornwall
This book is printed on acid-free paper responsibly manufactured from sustainable forestry in which at least two trees are planted for each one used for paper production.

Contents

About the author

DR MARK FORSHAW is a Senior Lecturer in Psychology at Leeds Metropolitan University. He has previously worked at Coventry University and the University of Manchester and has wide research interests within the realm of health psychology. He has published articles on topics as diverse as psychological aspects of physiotherapy and on deafness in newborns, and spends a great deal of his time involved in a number of book-writing projects. He is a Chartered Health Psychologist and an Associate Fellow of the British Psychological Society. His pastimes include writing poetry, abstract painting and world cinema.

Preface

This book should, I hope, be a useful source of information for two groups of people: those wishing to learn more about headaches and migraine because they are prey to them, and those who are simply interested. I would not, and cannot, claim that this book will definitely lead to a cure for your headaches. It might, but there are no guarantees. The information provided here may help you to identify possible causes of your condition and can certainly help you to find out more. Doctors sometimes disagree about the causes of headaches and have a range of opinions on the best ways to cure or ameliorate them. However, those in the medical professions are working hard to come to a conclusion, to establish some 'hard facts' about headaches and their treatment. What you must appreciate are the difficulties associated with this work. There are, it seems, thousands of plausible, potential causes of headaches, and it is sometimes almost impossible to pin-point them in any given individual. We all differ in so many ways, and our lifestyles are diverse. As a health psychologist, I am only too aware of how tiny differences between people can add up to a great deal. When doctors tell you honestly that they do not know the cause of your condition, they are not failing you but simply expressing the huge problem they face when diagnosing and treating many of the illnesses that have a strong psychosocial component. Headaches are not like broken bones; they are as much associated with your mind as with your body. This doesn't mean that headaches are imaginary but that they are *affected*, and sometimes caused by or made worse, by the mind and by our behaviour. If you read the 'Research in Brief' boxes in this book you will understand more what is meant by this.

It is possible to read this book without reading the Research in Brief boxes. They are provided for those readers who are interested in the research that has been conducted by academics and practitioners aiming to find out more about headaches and migraines. There is a mixture of psychological and medical research outlined in Research in Brief. No knowledge of medicine or psychology is required of the reader, although if you are not curious about research into headaches then feel free to ignore these boxes. You can even return to them later, since they largely can stand on their own.

The case histories that you will find in this book are true accounts written by 'expert patients', people who really understand what it is like to experience headaches and migraines. Many of you will empathise with their stories. I have edited them lightly, where necessary, but they remain largely as they were written. My profound thanks are extended to those people who provided these fascinating insights. For a host of reasons they will remain anonymous; however, they were asked to adopt a pseudonym of their own choosing, and their ages are correct.

One note is necessary on terminology. As far as possible I have retained the common medical terminology throughout this book, with explanations where necessary. I would rather do this than use terms that a person might then repeat to his or her doctor, only to create confusion. Similarly, I want people to be able to understand what their doctor says to them about their headaches. There is a special word for a person who experiences migraines, namely *migraineur* (bear in mind that when you are sure you are talking about a woman then, strictly speaking, this should be *migraineuse*). I have adopted this frequently throughout. To my knowledge, there is no single word for a person who has headaches.

As a psychologist, my main professional interest is in understanding the nature of the interaction between the mind and the body. We speak of 'psychogenic' phenomena: those things that are created by the mind. In the early stages of researching and writing this book, I was aware that I was fortunate enough never to have experienced a migraine. I say fortunate, but in some ways experience is everything. However, within months of beginning to write this book an event occurred which is relevant to recount here. One morning, while getting ready for work, I noticed a blotch of light in the right-hand side of my visual field. It grew, becoming more and more like a zig-zag arc of scintillating light, rainbow coloured, which slowly moved further and further across to the right, until it eventually disappeared after around 15 minutes. It was a classic pre-migrainal sign, of course. Thankfully, I did not develop a migraine. Thankfully also, I knew enough to be calm about this, rather than afraid. Some people would say that this was entirely imagined by me, but it certainly felt real. It has since happened two or three times, and a pattern has begun to emerge: on each occasion I was in a period of considerable stress. In fact, ironically, the work on this book contributed to that stress. Perhaps the aura was a warning sign to take things a little easier. I regard myself as very lucky to have had those signs, because they have helped me to understand migraines a little bit more and have helped me to put my work and stress into perspective. However, I am aware of the vast difference between what I have experienced and the 'hell' through which many migraineurs, and those people subject to chronic or cluster headaches, have to live. I am in awe of their courage.

About this book

In the first chapter, the differences between headaches and migraines are outlined, to help you to recognise which is which. In Chapter 2, differences between headache types are discussed and how these affect some kinds of people more than others, women more than men, and so on. In Chapter 3, real accounts of headaches from sufferers help us to understand what each of the main types of headache feels like. In our longest chapter, the fourth, the common and rarer causes of headaches and migraine are catalogued. The fifth chapter deals with the short- and long-term consequences of having headaches, and in Chapter 6 there is an outline of treatments. Following that, there is a section on finding help and further information, and a checklist to help you to work out what kind of headache you might be experiencing. It is possible to read the chapters of the book in any order, although they have been put together in an order that is probably the best if you want a coherent 'story' of headaches.

Acknowledgements

In preparing, researching and writing this book a number of people have proved invaluable, and I thank them warmly. Ann Rush, previously of the Migraine Action Association, graciously put me in touch with Dr Manuela Fontebasso. I would like to thank Manuela heartily for her time and patience in reading through a draft of this book, checking it for medical accuracy. She did so carefully yet quickly – something, which I appreciate, must have been quite a task given her other, substantial commitments. Kim Boccato is also to be thanked for a preliminary proof-reading of the text at short notice. Dr Jane Ogden, the series editor, was highly supportive of my interest in writing this book, and Dr Viv Ward and Deborah Egleton at Wiley have proved to be impeccable editors. Finally, I express my gratitude to Amanda Crowfoot for her love and moral support, as always.

Headache or migraine, acute or chronic?

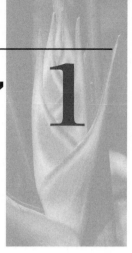

Most of the time, it is possible to work out whether someone has a headache or a migraine. There are usually clear differences between the two, as you will see from this chapter.

Headaches differ in both intensity and in type, or quantity and quality if you like, which means that two headaches of similar type but differing in intensity can end up in two different categories. However, as with many things in life, there can be confusions in the grey areas where one category meets another. (Could anyone say exactly when they stop liking someone and start loving them, or exactly when day becomes night?) To confuse the issue further, within the category of 'headache' there are many sub-types. In addition, how long you have them for can influence whether a doctor perceives you to be a victim to either acute or chronic headaches.

Some people will often say they have a migraine when actually they do not. Similarly, some people with a migraine think that they simply have a 'bad headache'. Hopefully, reading this book will help a few of these people to get a clearer picture. Sometimes, knowing what is wrong is half the way to a solution.

It is not possible to divide up headaches clearly into different categories without any overlap or blurring. The nature of the subject matter precludes this. There are even a number of interchangeable words for ordinary headache – *cephalodynia, cephalalgia* and *encephalalgia* – and if you ever look at your medical notes, you might find that some of these terms have been used. Don't be worried if you become a little confused by the fact that descriptions of apparently different headache types seem similar at times. This is unavoidable, since they do genuinely overlap. Imagine if someone asked you to describe yourself in a few words. Whatever words you chose would also be reasonably accurate words to describe millions of other people, and so it is with headaches. They differ in type as well as intensity, but trying to condense the complicated experiences of individuals into some type of common description means that some of the accuracy is lost. Headaches differ so much from person to person that there are bound to be problems when we try to outline what makes a 'typical' tension headache, for example. However, there is some common ground, as you will see. Another thing to consider is that someone can occasionally have more than one type of headache at the same time. Doctors are accustomed to seeing patients who have both migraines and tension-type headaches.

Primary or secondary?

If you read about headaches and migraines, there is a good chance that you will come across the terms 'primary' or 'secondary'. In fact, your doctor might even use these terms. Most people – that is, around 90 per cent – have primary headaches. These are headaches which exist entirely on their own and are not related to any other medical condition. Quite simply, they are headaches that are not really a sign of any other underlying disease or illness. Secondary headaches, on the other hand, are related to other conditions, and they are known as 'secondary' because they are a 'secondary symptom'. These types of headache occur precisely because you have some other physical problem. For example, your headache may be the result of high blood pressure (hypertension) and people with diabetes can get headaches for the same reason. At first, a doctor might be unsure whether your headaches or migraines are caused by some other factor, and this is why he or she might do other tests to eliminate certain possibilities. Different people accept the diagnosis of primary or secondary headaches in different ways. For some people, there is a relief associated with knowing that their headaches are primary. They are happy to know that there is no underlying cause, no illness lurking in the background. For other people, this is too vague, and they would actually rather be told that their headaches are secondary because at least they then know what is wrong. They find it difficult to live with pain when the doctor cannot identify a clear reason for it. You might like to think about which type of person you are, especially if you are about to see your doctor to get your headaches checked out. Spend some time dwelling on your likely reactions to being told that your headaches are either primary or secondary. It's not self-indulgent to think about yourself now and then: it can help you to see who you are and what you are.

Headache or migraine?

Strictly speaking, a migraine is a form of headache (it is even referred to as a 'migraine headache'). However, because it is rather a special form, it is usually seen as separate, is given its own name, and people study it specifically. It is probably easier to begin with defining a migraine first, since headaches tend to be defined as anything other than a migraine.

Migraines tend to be on one side of the head only (they are *unilateral*). Many people know that a migraine is going to occur because they might feel irritable, unduly tired, crave certain foods or even yawn excessively for hours or even days before it begins. This period is called the 'prodrome'. Some people then experience an aura which tends to begin just before the migraine itself. This aura is often in the form of a visual disturbance. We can divide migraineurs into two types based upon the aura, and these two different kinds of migraine were previously known as 'common' or 'classic'. Although some doctors will still use these terms, they have now been officially abandoned in favour of 'migraine without aura' and 'migraine with aura'. Most migraines are not accompanied by an aura. A migraine aura can come in a number of forms, which can include a strange taste in the mouth, or smelling something that is not there, or even a sense of feeling detached from reality. Most commonly, there is some visual disturbance, often a rainbow-like arc which moves across the visual field (a term we use to describe what you can see when your eyes are open). Sometimes it is in the form of flashing lights before your eyes, called *phosphenes*. (Don't confuse this with what can happen when you suddenly stand up after having been bending down for some time, although it can appear to be the same.)

Although the aura can last for some time, it is usually something that develops gradually over about 5 to 20 minutes and usually lasts up to an hour. As it can overlap with the migraine itself, it is not always something that comes before, and only before, the migraine. For those people who have an aura, it can be a useful warning to enable them to can take a painkiller or seek out a quiet place before the migraine starts properly.

Migraines tend to be pulsating: they throb. The pain is very strong, and you will commonly feel sick, or perhaps even vomit. You are likely to be unable to withstand strong light, often just normal dim daylight, and you are possibly equally averse to sound. In addition, moving around, especially moving the head, can make migraines much worse. So, a person with a migraine is typically someone who feels the need to go to bed, seeking quiet, darkness, and inactivity. Some people can go to sleep with a migraine and wake up fine, whereas others can wake up still in pain. Generally, a migraine lasts from about 4 to 72 hours. If you go to sleep with a migraine and wake up with it, you would count your time asleep in its duration.

A headache, on the other hand, can be any pain in the head which is not a migraine. However, certain head-pains are not headaches. Toothache, for instance, is an obvious example, but sometimes toothache can cause pain in the head which is actually felt on the skull. This kind of confusing pain is known to doctors as referred pain (because it is being 'referred' from one part of the body to another). One useful way to tell whether you have a headache that is actually toothache is by tapping your teeth, one by one, with your finger. You have to be brave, because when you find the right tooth you will get a lot of pain. In fact, anything going wrong with the head area, such as an ear infection, can create a pain that is quite indistinguishable from a headache.

The most common true headache is the tension-type, which might be called a 'stress headache' by your doctor. Stress headaches are the ordinary everyday headaches that most people have every now and then, and they are usually brought on by some kind of muscular stress in the neck or shoulders. This type of headache can be the result of psychological stress, because stressed people hunch up and tense their back and neck muscles even if they are not aware of it. Tension-type headaches can last for days but are often relieved quite quickly if the person takes some aspirin or other painkiller. They tend to be all over the head, commonly feeling as if someone has put a tight band around the head. They do not tend to be associated with other symptoms, unlike migraine, although some sickness can occur. When people get other symptoms, they are usually individuals who also suffer from migraines.

Cluster headaches are rarer than migraines or tension-type headaches, but are still the third most common. If you have a cluster headache, you will probably be in intense pain in your eye socket, and the eye might be red and weeping. The terrible pain will last up to a few hours and go away again only to return later. This can sometimes be mistaken for trigeminal neuralgia, where you experience shooting pain up one side of the face, and the skin of the cheek is often highly sensitive to touch. Cluster headaches are very distressing for their sufferers, and the pain is so strong that they can do nothing during an attack other than try to cope with it. Getting on with household chores or watching TV are generally not options. The pain is too intense to allow you to do everyday things, and sufferers often dance or pace around to try to relieve the agony.

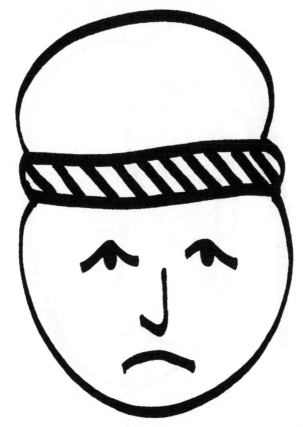

A headache which feels like a tight band is around the head is likely to be tension-type, rather than a migraine.

Elsewhere in this book you will learn about many other types of headaches, indeed doctors have identified as many as 150 different types based upon their many causes. Although it is a large number, it is because there are so many reasons why a headache can develop. In many ways, your head is the most important part of your body. Most of the things you do are controlled by the brain directly or indirectly, and so it is not surprising that there are so many ways in which the head can 'go wrong'. If you break your ankle, you get pain in the ankle. When something related to the head goes wrong, you can get a headache. Since the head is in charge of most things, including the way your ankle functions, something wrong in any part of your body can, in theory, give rise to a headache. Perhaps you can see why doctors have such a difficult job to do when working out why you have a headache.

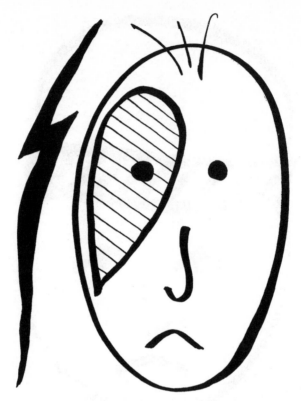

Striking, intense, pain down one side of the face could be cluster headache.

Acute (episodic) or chronic?

This is a tricky question for doctors. The first time anyone has a headache (probably as a baby) it is obviously an acute headache, because there is no history attached to it. Most of us go through life having occasional headaches and they are generally seen as individual acute episodes (you will also find that doctors talk of 'episodic' versus 'chronic' headaches and migraines). Similarly, if someone has an outburst of eczema once every 10 years we would also regard this as acute. As you can see, therefore, the acute/chronic distinction is really about the frequency of occurrence of something, not its strength, and not even that it recurs. Our difficulties arise when we try to pin down exactly some borderline between acute and chronic headaches, or indeed other conditions, because that is very difficult to do. We all know how much people argue about the age of consent, for instance. In the UK, for some things, you are an adult at 18; for other things you are considered able to make your own decisions at 16; and you can drive a car at 17. In other countries, the ages for the same 'abilities' are different. Furthermore, there will always be people who are more mature at 15 than others are at 18. Similarly, with headaches, you will find that what one doctor calls a series of acute episodes, another will believe to be a chronic condition. The general guidelines on defining headaches come from the International Headache Society. They specify that a chronic tension-type headache is one that occurs for 15 or more days each month for at least six months. Of course, here is our problem. If a headache occurs for 14 days each month for six months, it does not meet the criterion. While such guidelines are helpful, they do not always cover every possibility, and so the doctor rightly has room for discretion and judgement.

There is no equivalent specification of time for the diagnosis of chronic migraines produced by the International Headache Society. Usually, people who have migraines tend to have them regularly over a long period of time, and so, in a sense, almost all are chronic migraine sufferers.

Box 1.	Myths about headaches and migraines.

People commonly get the wrong idea about headaches and migraines. Lots of myths contain a grain of truth which is why they can sometimes flourish; but a grain of truth is not the same as a fact.

- **Headaches and migraines are excuses for people who don't want to work.** It is true that people sometimes take days off work because they claim to have a headache or migraine, and sometimes they are lying. However, some people also say that they have food poisoning when they have no such thing. The vast majority of people who have severe headaches or migraine are genuine and are in considerable pain.

- **Headaches and migraines are all in the mind; they are just psychological.** There is a psychological component to headaches, and it is true that people can think themselves into a headache. However, most headaches and migraines are very real, and we can even use complicated scanning techniques to prove it.

- **Headaches and migraines are just something people have to put up with.** If this were true, why would so many doctors be ▶

working so hard to find cures? There are things that can be done to help, and no one should simply grin and bear it.

- **Strong headaches are the same as migraines.** No, they are definitely not. As you will see from this book, although there are similarities, there are also differences. Sometimes strong headaches can be just as awful, if not more so, than migraines, but they are not the same thing.

- **Headaches are nothing to worry about.** Headaches are *usually* nothing to worry about – that much is true. However, headaches – especially if they are very sudden and strong or if they are occurring regularly – can sometimes be a sign of some other ailment that needs to be investigated. If in doubt, see your doctor.

- **Headaches are serious and a sign of something really terrible.** Although some headaches can be serious, most headaches are not.

- **You shouldn't bother your doctor with a headache.** If you have any concerns or questions, see your doctor. When you have worries or doubts about your health, you should talk to your doctor. Don't be afraid to approach your doctor as he or she would rather have you check things out than leave them until they become more difficult to treat. A stitch in time saves nine.

- **Migraines are a women's thing.** Mostly, in statistical terms, this is true, especially when you count menstrual migraines, but there are lots of men who would tell you that it is also a men's thing.

- **Doctors know everything there is to know about headaches and migraines as they are uncomplicated and easy to treat.** This is far from the truth. Doctors know a lot about these conditions, just as they know a lot about many things, such as pain, viral illnesses, and so on. However, there is a great deal still to be discovered and treatments are still being formulated. Patients may try many treatments, in conjunction with their doctor, before their best individual treatment is found.

Points to note

- Headaches are complicated things. Sometimes the signs and symptoms of different kinds of headache overlap, but generally it is possible to diagnose particular headaches if care is taken.
- Primary headaches are those which are themselves the main medical problem. Secondary headaches occur as a symptom of some other medical condition.
- Migraines tend to be on one side of the head and are usually throbbing. They make people hypersensitive to light and/or sound. Sometimes they are associated with an aura.
- Tension-type headaches are relatively steady, rather than throbbing, and are frequently based around the temples or feel like a tight band around the head. They are chronic if they occur for half of the days in a month for six months or more.
- Toothache, eye strain, or tension in the shoulders or neck can sometimes be confused for a headache.

Who has headaches and migraines?

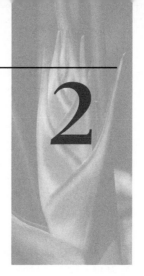

2

This chapter is dedicated to outlining who is likely to experience headaches of various types and who is or is not likely to be a migraineur.

We can begin this chapter with a simple statement. Anyone can have headaches and migraines, regardless of their age, background, medical history, and so on. However, such a simple statement is not particularly helpful, and we must remember that the person's condition introduces probabilities. Just because someone is unlikely to experience something does not mean that it will not happen. On the other hand, even a favourite can lose a race, regardless of the odds. In other words, there are trends to be observed, but they are only trends and there are always exceptions to the rule. For example, if you are a man, don't think that something cannot affect you because it mainly affects women. The only exception to this is that you cannot get problems related to women's reproductive systems, of course!

Famous migraineurs

We sometimes have a tendency to think of many medical conditions as a modern thing. We can forget that many people had headaches and migraines long before doctors had a name for them or knew anything about their true causes. Some key figures in history have been reputed to suffer from migraines (or headaches of some sort, since we cannot be sure without travelling back in time). These include Napoleon Bonaparte and Elvis Presley, both of whom managed to combine a fairly successful career with their medical condition, showing, perhaps, that headaches need not take over your life. One fascinating historical figure who, it is claimed, had migraines, is a nun named Hildegard von Bingen. She died around 800 years ago and is famous for many things, including her composition of religious music. She also experienced 'visions' throughout her life, which were interpreted as visitations from angels and other holy phenomena. Of course, it's not for us to say that this interpretation is not the truth. However, some now argue that the visions match very closely the visual disturbances found among migraineurs, such as the scintillating aura. Hildegard saw arcs of light in front of her eyes, like the wings of angels. Of course, to the non-religious, this bears a striking similarity to a symptom of migraine. She saw showers of stars, which can be interpreted today as phosphenes (which many people occasionally experience, not just migraineurs). Our evidence for this comes from the illustrations and descriptions that she left behind in her writings. To a modern doctor, the parallels between her visions and the signs of migraine are startling. To read more about Hildegard von Bingen, try Oliver Sacks's book *Migraine*, or try an internet search for Hildegard herself.

Men and women

Migraines are mainly experienced by women – in fact they affect three times more women than men. Obviously, this figure is added to by the fact that some women have migraines which are associated with their menstrual cycle. These can take two forms, the true menstrual migraine and the menstruation-related migraine. True menstrual migraines are caused, it is thought, by hormonal changes and can be treated by drugs similar to those in contraceptive pills. This type of migraine affects around 10 per cent of women and occurs on the first day of the menstrual cycle plus or minus two days. Therefore, they can occur as early as two days before the start of the cycle, or three days into it. (Of course, when a woman has a disrupted cycle this may be more difficult to determine.) True menstrual migraines are most likely to be migraines without aura.

Menstrual-related migraines, however, are more common (up to two-thirds of women claim that their periods can make migraines worse) and can happen at any time in the menstrual cycle, but they are often experienced at a particular point within the cycle, such as ovulation. Migraines can be part-and-parcel of general PMS and can be caused by a number of factors, including psychological factors such as stress. For some women, periods are very stressful: they may be painful or are perceived to be messy; they may make the women feel ill; or the women may also have problems that make the periods unpredictable. We know that stress contributes to migraines, and so it makes sense to assume that menstrual stress can lead to menstrual-related migraines. Tension-type headaches are also often commonly associated with menstruation. However, to complicate the issue, some women say that their migraines are less severe during menstruation!

Box 2. **Research in brief: menstrual-related migraines.**

Holm, Bury and Suda (1996) were interested in the relationship between menstruation, migraine and stress in women. They selected 12 women migraineurs and matched them with 12 other women who did not have migraines. In that way they could compare the normal effects of menstruation on stress with any interference in this relationship that might be related to migraines. They gave the migraine-prone women questionnaires on stress and coping, and asked them to complete a diary for a month, recording their headaches. It appeared, from their results, that at certain points on the menstrual cycle the women were less able to combat stress – that is, their coping strategies were not as good as the control group, and their migraines increased at these times. The relationship between stress and migraine varied, depending on the menstrual cycle itself. The researchers say that all of these factors interact with each other, so that when menstruating, women may experience more stress and therefore more migraines. Their psychological coping mechanisms are also affected. Thus, we can see that if we are to understand migraines in women we ought also to be ready to understand their menstrual patterns. We must remember, however, that this study only recorded one month of menstrual activity and with a rather small number of women. Psychologists always try to have rather larger numbers of volunteers in their studies so that their findings are representative of the population as a whole.

During pregnancy, another time of great hormonal activity, a proportion of women claim that their headaches or migraines are less severe, but there are some who feel that they are worse. This shows that we cannot simply explain migraine in terms of what is happening in the body, since roughly the same thing happens to all women when they are pregnant, at least in terms of chemical and physical changes. Rather, it seems that bodies, and minds, can react differently to the same events. What causes a migraine in one person can, theoretically, prevent it in another. Migraine can have its first occurrence during pregnancy, especially if it is associated with aura, and is more likely to be experienced by women who have menstrual migraines.

Tension-type headaches are commonly experienced by both men and women, of course. In fact, virtually everyone will have at least one at some point in life. Most people will have a number of tension-type headaches each year, and anything up to one a week, on average, can be normal even for a relatively healthy person. As with migraines, they are more common in women than in men, but not dramatically so. Up to 90 per cent of women experience tension-type headaches, and up to 70 per cent of men. To many people they are a normal part of life, and taking aspirin or some other painkiller gives relief until the next occurrence. For some others, however, they can be a lifetime problem.

Cluster headaches are mainly a male thing (about 85 per cent of them being experienced by men), which can create some confusion over diagnosis in this type of headache. Doctors can confuse this headache with many other things, so if you are a woman with a cluster headache it is less likely that your doctor will immediately spot the problem and make an accurate diagnosis. Doctors work on probabilities; they match your symptoms with what something *probably* is, which is why they sometimes do not think that a lump on a young woman's breast is likely to be cancer; it is simply that it is not likely to be cancer because younger women tend not to get breast cancer, although, of course, some do.

Sexually-related headaches are, despite what you might imagine, experienced more by men than by women. We have all heard of the 'not tonight, I have a headache' scenario, but in our sexist world we tend to think this is an excuse used by women to abate their lustful partners. In fact, most sexual headaches are caused by sex itself, and are far more common in men than in women (men outnumbering women four to one). These headaches commonly occur at the start of sexual activity, or at the point of orgasm. If you consider the nature of arousal, it is not surprising that when the blood starts pumping through the veins the likelihood of a headache can increase. Don't be afraid of telling your doctor about sexual headaches. The doctor cannot help you or give you advice if he or she does not have the whole story. No matter what you tell your doctor, even if it is very private and embarrassing for you, it will all have been heard before.

A political note

Throughout history, women have been treated differently from men, not only in society as a whole but in specific aspects of life. Dealings with the medical profession are not exempt from this. There is a great deal of evidence to show that doctors are sometimes more likely to assume that women are more neurotic and anxious than men. In the early days of medicine, it was believed for instance that the uterus was responsible for making people neurotic. Therefore, using this reasoning, only women were capable of being unduly anxious. The Greek word for womb was borrowed and adapted to describe this psychiatric condition: hysteria. We have moved on a lot from this, but some doctors are still a little sexist and one should be aware of this. There is some modern evidence that stereotyping still pervades certain aspects of the medical profession.

When a woman visits the doctor, she is more likely than a man to have her complaint dismissed. This is an important issue when considering headaches because we know that headaches can have a significant psychological component. It is only too easy for a doctor to think that your headaches are 'imaginary' or trivial if he or she happens to believe that women are neurotic and tend to worry about every little thing. Therefore, if you are female you may have to try and try again before your doctor will take your headaches seriously and investigate them properly. It is unlikely, of course, because, most doctors are fair and professional, but subtle forms of sexism pervade our lives and we need to be sensitive to them. Don't make the mistake of thinking that only male doctors are likely to have such negative perceptions of women. Female doctors are probably just as likely to hold on to sexist stereotypes.

Headaches through the lifespan

Headaches in babies are almost impossible to identify unless we use expensive scanning techniques. A baby who cries far too much could be experiencing persistent headaches, but most of the time we never know. Only when they are old enough to indicate the source of their pain can we properly begin to investigate the issues. Migraines are the most common type of headache in small children, although other types do occur, and equal numbers of boys and girls tend to be affected. The sex difference only really starts to show properly when children are in their teenage years. The vast majority of headaches in children are relatively harmless, so if your child has headaches you should not worry unduly, but should always contact your doctor in any case since it is always best to have children's health complaints checked out thoroughly. Children who are susceptible to headaches of any type tend to have some kind of sleep disturbance. Quite often the headaches keep them awake at night, and they are then quite tired during the day. This can be a sign to the parents that headaches are to blame for their children's health problems.

Just as with adults, there are many reasons why children might have headaches. There are, however, a few additional reasons for children, in particular, being affected. Hormonal changes in puberty can be a cause. Children are also more susceptible to additives in food, such as colourings and preservatives. However, one commonly overlooked cause, which is actually more important in the lives of most children, concerns the amount of time they spend each day in front of screens of some sort. They play computer games for hours, and when they are not doing this they might be watching television. The resulting eye strain, not to mention the postural strains caused by being hunched over a computer monitor, can lead directly to headaches. Add this to the fact that children attend school, where they also use computers, and spend a lot of the day reading and writing, and you have the perfect recipe for headaches. Children often do not notice that they are straining to see things, so make sure that their eyes are checked by an optician at regular intervals.

Headaches in children are not uncommon, and when migraines occur they can often take a very strange form: an abdominal migraine. This is experienced as a pain in the stomach rather than the head, and sometimes a child feels pain in both areas. Abdominal migraine, however, is much rarer in adults. Parents can be very cautious about their children claiming to have stomach pains or headaches because it can be a common excuse to stay away from school. Be sensitive to your child's circumstances, and try to sort out the real headaches from the pretend ones.

HELPFUL TIPS! HELPFUL TIPS! HELPFUL TIPS! HELPFUL

If your child only reports headaches during school times, and never at weekends or during holidays, then there is a good possibility that something else is going on. Look carefully for the patterns and, if you find them, speak to your child's teachers about what happens at school.

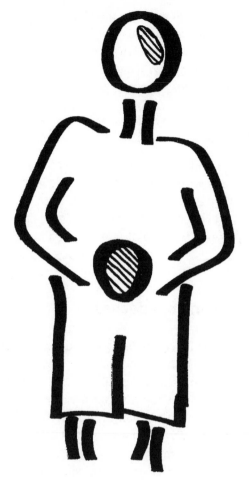

In children especially, migraines can be felt in the stomach area as well as the head.

It is commonly found that people report fewer migraines when they reach their fifties and that cluster headaches and tension-type headaches also decrease in frequency. However, headaches for other reasons become more common, unfortunately. As we age, we become more susceptible to cardiovascular disease and diabetes, for example, which are associated with headaches. The sad truth is that headaches of one sort or another affect us all of our lives, and it's only the *type* of headache that changes over time. We are more prone to arthritis as we grow older and this too can create headaches, especially if the arthritis is in the bones of the neck.

One particular problem in people in their later years is temporal arteritis, sometimes known as giant cell arteritis. It affects more women than men and tends to start after the age of 50, but is most common when people are in their seventies. It involves inflammation of the arteries around the head, and doctors are not sure why this happens.

HELPFUL TIPS! HELPFUL TIPS! HELPFUL TIPS! HELPFUL

If you are over 50 and have a very tender scalp around the temples – perhaps with a headache which is worse at night and feels particularly painful in the cold – you should speak to your doctor and report these symptoms. He or she can then conduct further tests to see if you are affected by temporal arteritis.

Medical history and headaches

If you visit your doctor with a complaint about headaches, he or she will look at your medical records to find any reasons as to why you are experiencing them. If the doctor does not do so, he or she might miss some important information. For instance, if you are diabetic or hypertensive, then this could explain the problem. Of course, if you have had many health problems over the years, your records could be extensive. In fact, any doctor will tell you that some patients have records that contain hundreds of pages. If this is the case, your doctor may find it very difficult to check all of them and may miss some important information. This is why some self-research may help. No one knows your medical history better than you. Therefore, spend some time thinking about the health problems you have now, or have had in the past, and do some reading about headaches. If your doctor is unable to explain your complaint, then you should suggest anything that your own research has uncovered. This is not telling your doctor how to do his or her job but is helping your doctor to solve your problem. We have moved far away from the days when the doctor was seen as an absolute expert and the patient a complete novice. Most models of health care today strongly incorporate the view that diagnosis and treatment are part of a process of negotiation and cooperation between health-care professionals and their patients. If you car breaks down, you tell the mechanic what happened, rather than expecting him to simply work out what is wrong with the vehicle. So when you see your doctor, produce the facts he or she needs to help you.

HELPFUL TIPS! HELPFUL TIPS! HELPFUL TIPS! HELPFUL

You might have had an injury to your neck or spine as a child. Although it may have healed many years ago, it could be the cause of headaches.

Box 3. Research in brief: self-efficacy.

Psychologists have spent considerable time researching a concept called self-efficacy. Basically, it concerns the faith that people have in themselves to be able to do things. If people have high self-efficacy they have confidence in themselves. Those with lower self-efficacy generally do not feel as if they can do much about their situation because they feel they lack the necessary abilities or skills. People vary widely in their self-efficacy, and this might have consequences for many aspects of their lives, including health and illness.

Marlowe (1998) investigated the idea that self-efficacy might affect how people cope with stress, and how this might, in turn, affect how they experience headaches. He interviewed 120 headache sufferers, aged from 17 to 65 years. In addition, these volunteers also kept track of their headaches and stressful events in their lives over a period of 28 days. In 114 of these people (95 per cent), there was a clear relationship between stressful events and headaches. The more stressful events that occurred, the more headaches were experienced. What is interesting is how this interacted with self-efficacy. In people with high self-efficacy, the relationship between stressful events and headaches was weakest, but for those individuals with low self-efficacy there was a strong relationship between headaches and stress. This tells us that when people have faith in themselves they can fight off headaches when stress occurs. When people lack this confidence, stress is given free reign to lead to headaches. This is important because self-efficacy is something that can be changed. If a psychologist can work with people to increase their confidence in themselves to defeat stress and cope with it, then it is possible that they can be helped to break the link between stressful ▶

episodes in life and the onset of a headache. You cannot get rid of stress, since it is a normal part of every person's life, but it might be possible to work on our reactions to stress, and our self-beliefs.

Occupation

If you work in a high-stress occupation (for example, teaching, some types of business, and prison work) you are more likely to experience tension-type headaches and, possibly, migraines. There is a clear link between stress and most types of headache, and so your work-life can be a clear cause of this and other medical conditions. You probably cannot change your work. You are unlikely to be able to stop unpleasant things happening, and you are possibly not able to have much influence on your workload. For most of us, work is something that is handed to us, rather than something that we create for ourselves. Most of the time, there is only one thing that you can change, and that is your attitude to work. Stress is always perceived. If you do not perceive stress, then it is not there. Of course, it is very easy for someone to suggest that you should simply stop feeling stressed. There are, nevertheless, things you can do to counter stress, such as finding time to relax. In cases where your health is really at risk, a psychologist can help you to redefine your stress.

People who work with toxic materials as part of their job may be more susceptible to headaches, especially if there is unavoidable contact with those substances. Although health and safety organisations monitor such exposure, we all know that accidents can and do happen, and, occasionally, people can become complacent and fail to follow the guidelines set out by the authorities. Headaches can, in theory, be triggered by any exposure to hazardous materials (most people have experienced a headache from painting a room in their house, for example) or even by lead absorbed through the skin. Therefore, if you are experiencing regular headaches, speak to your doctor about your work, and perhaps the person responsible for health and safety at your workplace.

Heredity

Many people naturally want to know if headaches and migraines are passed down in families. The answer to this is simple: yes and no. There is *some* evidence of heredity, but there is by no means a perfect relationship between headaches and genetics. If you have no history of migraine in the family it does not mean that you will not experience migraines; it is simply less likely. If both your parents have migraines, you may not have them at present, but it is highly probable that you will suffer them eventually. This can be due to a number of reasons. If your migraines are of the allergic type, then you might have inherited a gene that makes you allergic to the same thing as one or both of your parents. But it is often difficult to work out what we can blame on genetic inheritance and what we can blame on upbringing. Psychologists have spent decades debating the so-called nature–nurture hypothesis. Not everything is due to genes. Sometimes, we learn things from our parents, regardless of genes. Stress, which is heavily involved in all types of headache, is something we cannot avoid because the world is full of things that can stress us. Some people cope very well with stress, and life's problems seem to be 'like water off a duck's back' to them. Other people do not have those coping skills, and are strongly affected by certain events. Coping skills are something that we teach our children, even when we are not trying. Children often emulate us and pick up tips and hints. They learn how to behave from us. If they see us responding badly to stress, they can learn to respond badly too. Children can therefore pick up their parents' habits, and if poor coping leads to greater stress and greater stress leads to headaches in the parents, it is quite likely that a similar pattern will be observed in the children when they grow up.

Race and culture

There is no current evidence to suggest that different 'races' of people have different types of headache, although there could easily be differences between people based on their culture. Coping styles can differ across cultures, types of stress experiences can vary and, most obvious of all, eating habits differ. As a simple example, Chinese food can be high in monosodium glutamate (MSG), a chemical which, it has been claimed, can lead to headaches. Irrespective of whether you are ethnic Chinese or not, eating a lot of Chinese food could contribute to a greater incidence of headaches. We are currently in a position where cross-cultural studies of headaches have seldom been conducted and published, and so we can only guess at the differences between people based upon such things. What does seem to hold true, however, concerns the frequency of headaches in different, very broad, racial groups. Quite simply, white people seem to get more headaches. Headaches are less common in

African-Caribbean people or Asian people (in both the British and the American sense of the word). We are not sure why this is, but differences in frequency of occurrence have been observed.

Points to note

- Migraines affect more women than men.
- For some women, menstruation makes migraines worse, but it can also provide relief in others.
- Tension-type headaches affect men and women, but not equally. More women are affected than men, but the difference in proportion is not so marked as in the case of migraine.
- Cluster headaches mainly affect men.
- Headaches can occur right through the lifespan, although the reasons for having them might change.
- Working in high-stress occupations can be a factor in developing headaches.
- There is some genetic evidence that migraines run in families, but the link is not strong.

What do they feel like?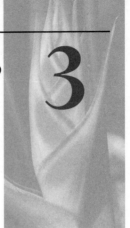

3

Most of this chapter is taken up with writings by
actual patients themselves – by the people who
know best what headaches and migraines
feel like.

The most important thing to point out is that even the word *headache* is something of a misnomer. Many people with headaches do not feel an ache at all. They feel burning pain, or sharp or stabbing pain, or something else. People with a pain in the head are simply reflecting the fact that we have, perhaps, chosen a bad word to represent headache. If we could start all over again, making new words, it might be better to say 'headpain', but we cannot change history. Psychologists try very hard to equate different people's experiences of pain, and construct words that we can all use and with which we all agree, but it is not an easy task. We all have our own ways of expressing things, and no two people are the same. So, when you read what people have to say about their headaches or migraines, remember that you will not always agree with them. Your experiences will be a little different.

In this chapter, you will read about what various types of headaches usually feel like. As with everything, there are exceptions to the rule, but it would take a lifetime to write a book about the unusual cases. Every possible type and cause of headache is not backed up with a personal account, simply because this book would consist of hundreds of pages were that to be so. The most common types are covered, however. The three most commonly diagnosed headaches are tension-type, migraine and cluster, and if you are having a headache it is probably one of these, and more probably one of the first two types.

Tension-type headaches

The following story shows how much a so-called normal headache, the tension-type, can easily be confused with migraine. In some cases, the main difference is in intensity rather than quality. In all of the talk about how terrible migraine can be, it is easy to forget the suffering that tension-type headaches, especially chronic ones, can bring.

❝The worst thing about tension headaches is that other people don't always have sympathy because they just think I am having normal, everyday headaches. It's true, I am, but I don't just get headaches like anyone else. I think they are worse, if only because I have them quite regularly.

I have headaches 10 to 20 times a month. What's more worrying is that I have had them for years and years at this level. They are a dull pain, and they just don't go away. They are worse when I move my head. Sometimes I feel sick, but not always, and once I also had blurred vision. At first I thought I had migraines, but the doctor ruled that out. When I get them, they can last two or three days, and I stop being able to concentrate on things because the constant pain just gets me down. Of late, the doctor has been suggesting that I might be depressed. The trouble is, he's right, but it's not that simple because I think that anyone who had had these headaches for so long would start to get depressed anyway. What I mean is that depressed people hate getting up in the morning, and so do I, but in my case it is often because I have gone to bed with a headache and woken up with a headache and know that I'm going to have a headache all day unless I am lucky and painkillers get rid of it, which they do sometimes but not always.

I have tried lots of things to deal with them, and painkillers seem to be the best, but I don't want to use them very often because I know they are not good for me in the long run. If my husband massages my shoulders I very often get relief, but it doesn't always last, and the headache can come back an hour after he stops. I have also tried Indian head massage, and that works too, but I can't get someone to do that to me at three in the morning when I can't sleep and my head feels like it is in a vice.

Anyone who has headaches like mine has a job on their hands. Sometimes, I wish I had migraines instead, because I know that they hurt more, but from what I have heard they don't take up as much of your time. The problem with chronic headaches is that it's hard to get anything done when half of your life is spent with pain in the head.❞

Sue, 55

Migraine with aura

Some people think they have influenza when they have a bad cold. Similarly, there are some individuals who claim that they have a migraine when it is simply a bad headache. Often, such people have never really experienced a true migraine. As can be seen from these stories, migraines involve lots of signs and symptoms which mean that they are generally much worse than a common headache.

Walter's story demonstrates the milder side of migraines. As you can see, he is lucky in that they seem to be well controlled and occur quite rarely. He is also fortunate because he is actually a psychologist, and therefore had books available from which he could find out about his condition, which no doubt helped him to put things into perspective. Of course, reading this book might provide that kind of reassurance for you, and there is a wealth of information out there if you know where to look. Later in this book there are pointers to help you to track down good information.

❝I have had migraines since childhood. I distinctly recall standing in a school dinner queue at about the age of 14 and experiencing the characteristic multicoloured snaking pattern of light slowly but surely arcing across the centre of my vision, eventually filling one whole half of my visual field. I thought it was odd, but never got scared as these things had happened many times before. After the visual disturbance there would usually be a period of about 30 minutes before a bad headache would kick in. It was not until I was about 22 that I came to understand that this was a classic migraine. I had been writing a paper at a computer and suddenly noticed that some of the words had 'disappeared'. Gradually the partial blindness got worse and the snaking pattern seemed to be the cause. I went and found a copy of the *Oxford Companion to the Mind* and looked up migraine. I found a perfect description of my experiences over the years. It also noted that the headache tended to kick in about 30 minutes after the visual disturbance, so I quickly took two paracetamol and managed to avoid the worst of the headache. These days I always do that and manage to keep the worst of it at bay. I have also noticed that my breathing appears to be 'strange' – gently laboured if that makes any sense – when I have a migraine. Breathing more slowly seems to help. Migraines are for me not a frequent thing – perhaps two or three a year.**❞**

Walter, 31

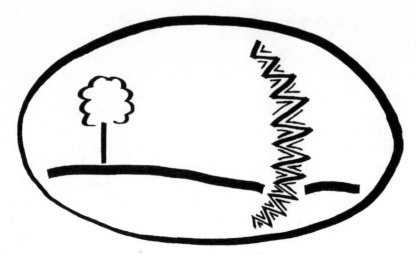

A common migraine aura involves a 'scintillating arc' of light moving its way across the field of view.

Migraines can have many causes, and many treatments. Hannah illustrates this very well in her account. Note that she relates her migraines to menstruation, so it is no coincidence then that she finds that chocolate can help to alleviate migraine. Many women turn to chocolate and other sweet foods during their period.

> **"**In my early teens I started to suffer with migraine-like symptoms on waking almost every Sunday morning. These were not accompanied by severe headaches, but I did feel very nauseous. I did not relate them to migraines until much more recently. In my mid-teens I suffered migraine-like headaches, when I had a temporary job in a poorly lit office, i.e. with flickering fluorescent lights.
>
> In my early twenties I suffered what I considered to be my first full-blown migraine. This started with a headache and nausea, which became progressively worse. I then suffered vomiting and started shaking violently and could not stand any light in my eyes.
>
> Since then, my migraines became quite a regular occurrence, particularly during menstruation. I recall having taken aspirin and paracetamol though do not believe these were actually of much assistance. The migraines would sometimes last for as little as a few hours but on occasions lasted for several days. Ten days was the longest duration. It never occurred to me to try to trace the cause at this stage.

In my thirties I was diagnosed with Irritable Bowel Syndrome, which, together with the migraines, was apparently due to stress. For a few years I was treated periodically with tranquillisers and beta-blockers. Though this did reduce the frequency and severity of both the migraines and the stomach cramps associated with the irritable bowel syndrome, I was very dissatisfied with the side-effects these drugs caused, so was determined not to rely on them permanently.

The breakthrough in determining the triggers of my migraines came only three-and-a-half years ago, in my mid-forties, when I suffered severe food poisoning. For over two weeks I was unable to eat anything without the symptoms recurring and it seemed that I would never get better. In desperation I visited an allergy-testing clinic. Though frowned upon by the medical profession this really was the turning point in my life. I was found to be intolerant to a wide range of food products, each of which was responsible for numerous ailments that I had been suffering for a number of years. After embarking on a diet which totally excluded all of these food products, not only did I lose the migraines and irritable bowel syndrome, but I also stopped suffering with hay fever and asthma. Unfortunately, it was too restrictive to stick to such an exclusive diet for too long a period and I still periodically suffer some of these symptoms now if I overdo the problem foods, but I have generally been a great deal better.

In the past, I have found that my migraines have been triggered by: artificial lights, dairy foods, sunlight, lack of sleep, dehydration, alcohol, menstruation, prolonged exposure to computer screens, food colourings (particularly tartrazine) and caffeine.

I have actually found that chocolate can help! This is perhaps the most controversial remedy, since it is generally considered a trigger. I sometimes get a real craving for chocolate during the early signs of a migraine. I don't believe it is just coincidence that the symptoms have disappeared on several occasions after eating a small bar of chocolate. **"**

Hannah, 49

In the following case, we learn that migraines can run in families, and that oversleeping can also be involved. Take note that the causes or triggers seem to have changed over the years for Charlotte. Something that seems to cause migraines today may not necessarily do so tomorrow. Keep track of your own migraine triggers, perhaps by maintaining a diary, and take note of any changes, informing your doctor from time to time if necessary.

❝I was diagnosed as a migraine sufferer as a child; my mother also being a sufferer noticed the symptoms and took me to see a doctor. I consider myself one of the luckier people as, in recent years, the headaches have been far less frequent than they once were. I remember very little about the pattern of my migraines from younger childhood, however, it was during my teenage years that I suffered the most and as such these experiences stay with me best.

Between the ages of about 11 and 16 I was guaranteed to get a migraine almost every Sunday morning. I often felt that this was due to the fact that I slept for far longer on Saturday nights than I did any other day of the week. The headache would get worse as the day went on, despite having taken painkillers as soon as I got up. Later in the day standing up from a seated position caused a tremendous dizziness which would often set me back down again, at these times the pain would increase suddenly too, so much so it felt like my head would explode at any minute. When I went to bed in the evening my head would be pounding while I was trying to get to sleep.

Waking up on the Monday morning I would lie in bed in the desperate hope that the headache would have gone, but inevitably it hadn't. I would spend the day functioning at half speed, finding concentration difficult, and eye strain easy to come by; the pain would last right through the day, sometimes accompanied by feelings of nausea. By the Tuesday morning the pain would have greatly reduced, and as the day went by, with the help of painkillers that now seemed to have some effect, the migraine would finally dissipate.

As I have got older the migraines have become a much rarer occurrence and, as far as I can tell, are not brought on by the amount of sleep I get. They can last for anything between 24 and 72 hours but always have the same characteristics: dizziness, nausea, pounding, high pressure, and increased eyestrain. I have never felt the need to bang my head against the wall like many people do, rather I feel I should be clutching the sides of my head in order to stop it from blowing up from the pressure, although I know that it can't happen. I also can't understand how all that pressure can be contained in my skull. I have tried almost every painkiller on the market but none of them even begin to work until they have built up; this tends to be around the time the pain is diminishing anyway.

I know that many people find their migraines triggered by things such as chocolate, stress, or menstruation in the case of many women, but these have never been triggers for me. I do feel that, earlier on, my migraines were down to too much sleep, but now I believe that they are due mainly to light. My eyes have always been very sensitive to light; I wear sunglasses almost all of the time, even in winter and at dawn and dusk. Having spoken to my optician about it she confirmed that I had high light sensitivity that could lead to headaches. 99

Charlotte, 23

Some migraines can alter your senses and temporarily take away your speech or vision, and it can be quite frightening when you do not know what is happening to you. It is quite natural to panic, especially when something seemingly dramatic happens, as shown in the following account.

66Typically, the first sign of an impending migraine is that printed text suddenly shimmers before my eyes, and it becomes very effortful to work out what a particular word says. This can be a brief experience, but it's a warning sign not to carry on reading. There are slight disturbances on the periphery of vision, but not really the 'aura' that is sometimes described. More typically, the edges of vision become slightly 'fogged', and there can be the impression of faint objects floating through my field of vision. This produces the strange compulsion to follow them by moving my head. This can produce a similar effect to a dog chasing its tail. Speech production, too, can suffer, and I can become unable to produce coherent speech. Fortunately, the severity of this declined with time, and has now largely disappeared. A numbness in my right hand usually occurs as well. It's difficult to explain to anyone who hasn't had a migraine just how painful it is. It is much more of a 'pain in the head' than a 'bad headache'. The pain is constant and throbbing and can produce nausea although, again, this has greatly reduced over the years.

The only thing to do is to take some painkillers and lie down in a very dark, very quiet place and try not to think about anything. The headache can continue for a couple of hours during which it is impossible to sleep; a migraine would be much more tolerable if one was able to sleep through it. After a migraine attack, I can feel 'washed-out' and drained for a couple of days, but this is sometimes followed by a period of euphoria. I don't know why – it must be endorphins or something. I suppose when strange things are happening in my brain, I shouldn't be surprised at any of the effects. The problem with thinking about migraines in order to describe their effects is that this can produce one, so I'm going to stop now. **"**

Barnaby, 33

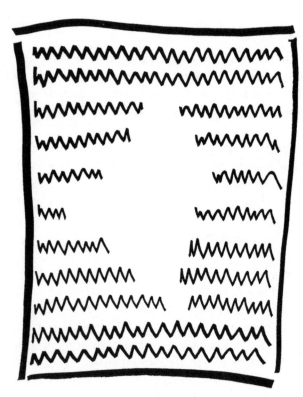

Visual disturbances during migraine can include disappearing or blurred text while reading.

The following account shows what happens to vision during a migraine. It can be particularly alarming for a child, of course, as in this story. Note that hearing seems to be involved here too.

❝My first migraine was probably the worst and the weirdest one I have experienced. I was 6 years old and at school at the time it started; at first it was like a constant dull thudding, then the nausea started (although I wasn't actually sick until I got home). The worst bit came after my mum had come to pick me up. I lost half my visual field, and I could not see the left side of anything, including faces. I also lost my sense of balance particularly on the left side of my body; in fact I lost most of the sensation down that side of my body. I could not judge distance or height. Sound was also amplified, and I ended up in hospital for a couple of hours. It took two days to recover from that one.

None of the others have been as spectacular as that one, and used to be associated with PMS (not every month but often enough). Now, however, they happen less often and I can usually tell if one is on the way and catch it before it gets too bad, however this has taken some time and occasionally it's either too late or the situation means I can't do anything about it. Most of my migraines start with a feeling of being in a waking dream; nothing feels real and sound becomes distorted, light sources become fuzzy (it's kind of like when you go swimming without goggles). If I catch it in time (by taking a tablet and going to bed) I don't

Migraines can involve seeing things that are not there, which can include dark flower-like blotches.

get a full-blown attack. However, I do still feel a little vulnerable the next day, and I am oversensitive to strong light, smells and loud noise. **"**

Lila, 23

The next account shows just how alarming a migraine can be when it has effects on the body and mind as a whole. In fact, in these more extreme cases, the person involved can even believe that he or she has experienced a stroke.

"I had quite severe headaches three weeks leading up to my first attack which started with a strange sensation of tingling 'pins and needles' in my left leg followed by numbness and then a feeling of total loss of control. My leg no longer moved the way I wanted it to; the only reason I knew where my leg was placed was by sight. The same sensation occurred in my left arm. I was only able to move my left arm by watching it, and often overshot the height I was trying to move it to; trying to lift my arm a couple of inches would result in it being over my head. The same sensation moved to my mouth, which became so numb that it became impossible to speak and I lost the ability to move my mouth to form letters and words. This experience was followed by severe headache and vomiting.

This experience happened four times within two weeks. The first two attacks were on the left side and the second two on the right. During the third attack I was fully aware of the order of events my migraine took and knew that there was nothing I could do to prevent it from happening. My body would be taken over by numbness for approximately 45 minutes, which would then be followed by vomiting. During my various stages of numbness several visual hallucinations occurred. I didn't suffer any flashing lights or colourful patterns, but while staring at a picture of a Spanish villa decorated with green plants I saw a bright green tortoise. I also realised that in 30 minutes' time I would be vomiting, so I decided to eat some food that was soft to make the experience a little bit more pleasurable (if there is such a thing!). I had to plan each step in my head from getting up from the sofa to walking into the kitchen. I found myself trying to put a potato into the toaster instead of the microwave; I had a sense of total disorientation.

After my third experience I was prescribed 80 mg of propranolol to be taken daily and have had just one incident of migraine since. **"**

Catherine, 20

Although the migraine in this case was alarming, with hallucinations, the solution was a simple one. Catherine was frightened by the experience, but all was well in the end. If you experience any symptoms like this, please do not panic. To be safe, however, you must contact a doctor.

Cluster headaches

These are predominantly a male burden, and are intensely painful. They are focused around one eye, usually on one side of the head only, and are sharp and stabbing. Before the headache, a 'warning' may occur, of aching on one side of the head and they often begin during sleep. They can last for less than an hour, but may exceed three or four hours. Sufferers may experience them many times a day for a period of weeks or months, and then they usually stop for some time. Indeed, they can go away forever, or for decades, only to return again. During the headaches the eye may stream and the nose might be blocked, which can lead to a mistaken diagnosis of hay fever, or some other allergy. Because they are more likely to occur during spring or autumn, they do seem like seasonal allergic reactions, hence the misdiagnosis. Furthermore, the fact that they are centred around the eye can lead doctors up a blind alley looking for causes in the eye itself or in the nerves in the neck and head.

The principal characteristic of this type of headache is the severity of the pain. It is often the worst pain the person has ever or will ever feel. It is so strong that during the headaches the sufferers may dance around to distract themselves from the pain, or hit themselves in the head. They may even repeatedly bang their heads against a wall or door post, although this is not to be recommended, of course. Because the pain is so strong, suicide is higher among people with cluster headaches than it is among people generally, or among migraineurs. Samuel tells his story:

"My cluster headaches first began when I was in my twenties. I noticed that alcohol tends to bring them on, so I don't touch it anymore, which can mean that I have to drive everyone around instead of being one of the party, as it were. When they happen, it is always on the left side of my face, and the pain is indescribable. I feel as if someone has put something into my face, like an injection of acid. If someone tore my eye out I am sure it would not be any less painful. My eye usually streams with tears; not just a little bit, but like I am crying. I feel like I can't do anything to take the pain away, and I don't know what to do or where to go. The pain takes over everything. I am disabled by it, and can't do anything but feel pain. I walk around and around, not knowing where to go; I want to be able to run away from it. I have resorted to hitting myself, because sometimes it can be distracting to do so. That's the main thing really, the need to find a distraction. I tend to get them in the winter, which made the doctor think I was having episodes of neuralgia, but I've had neuralgia when I was younger and I know the difference. Then the doctor thought it was sinusitis, but that too wasn't the answer. I now have oxygen from my doctor, and take it when I feel an attack coming on. It works most of the time. I have tried many other things to keep them in check, but for me the best thing has been the oxygen. It may sound odd, but I have heard that water helps a lot of people. They say it flushes out the system. I do try to drink mineral water as much as possible, because it can't do any harm.

I tend to get my cluster headaches for about three months at a time, with anything up to five attacks a day. Sometimes they are over in ten minutes, but sometimes they last for a couple of hours or more. When they happen, I can't do a thing. I just pray that they will stop. **"**

Samuel, 42

We have seen in this chapter the kinds of feelings people have about their headaches, and what the pain means to them and their lives. These stories show exactly why we need to take people seriously when they are experiencing headaches and migraines. Most of us get a little headache from time to time, but some people really suffer again and again, and those people deserve the best care that doctors can provide. Equally, they need all the support they can get from their families, friends and employers.

Points to note

- Even the same type of headache can feel different to different people.
- Headaches can affect everyone in varied ways.
- The symptoms of a migraine can be alarming, but usually the fear subsides considerably when a diagnosis is made.

The causes
of headache
and migraine

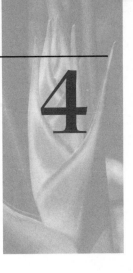

In this chapter, some of the common and rare causes of headaches are outlined. This, however, is not an exhaustive list.

Before you read this section, you must understand the following. This section of the book is not intended to allow you to make a diagnosis as to the cause of your headache. Only a doctor can really do that for you. This section is for information only. If you have any unusual symptoms, a strong headache, or one which has persisted for more than 24 hours, you are strongly advised to see your doctor.

One other point needs to be made. When you read this section, bear in mind something called **medical students' disease**. This is the psychological condition where studying or reading about illness and diseases can help to convince people that they are suffering from those ailments. It can affect anyone, not just those people who are anxious or hypochondriacal. When people read about something, they are susceptible to their imagination running wild. (It's quite similar to the way people often feel after watching a horror movie: they get jumpy and start to worry that an intruder is up the stairs or waiting for them in the wardrobe!) Medical students commonly experience this phenomenon. After learning that diabetes can be associated with intense thirst, they may start to feel thirsty. After studying diseases like arthritis, they start to notice the creaks and clicks in their joints. Learning about something makes you aware of it, but sometimes you become hyper-aware. The best way to avoid this problem is to **write down all of your symptoms before reading what follows**. If something is not on your list when you read further, it ought to help to put your mind at rest. Please do it now, before you read any further.

Just about *anything* can cause a headache (although the causes of migraine are somewhat more limited). In addition to things going wrong in the head or the body in general, headaches can stem from many of the things we eat

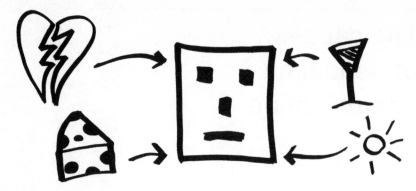

Stress, food, drink and light are all common causes of migraine.

or the things *missing* from our diet, disordered sleep, stress, noise, lighting, environmental pollution, overwork, and a myriad of other factors.

Common causes

Hangover

In some societies, arguably, most headaches occur as a result of 'the night before'. Drinking alcohol in large amounts poisons the body, and the result, for most people, is a headache the next day. Binge drinkers are especially prone to this, but moderate drinkers (a glass of wine with a meal each day, for instance) rarely experience a hangover. The headache that is felt from a hangover is due to inflammation of the meninges, a membrane covering the brain. The brain itself is not sore, since that is not possible, but the sac of skin surrounding it has lots of nerve cells that can respond to poisoning. The best way to avoid a hangover is by not drinking alcohol to excess, but if you do then drink large quantities of water before going to sleep. Take your time drinking the water, however, since gobbling down three pints of water and going straight to sleep is not advisable. The best advice is to drink water along with the alcohol, volume-for-volume. So, for every glass of wine you drink, have a glass of water. This will also help you to moderate your consumption of alcohol as you will find it more difficult to drink twice the amount of fluid! Bear in mind that it really should be water that you drink, not cola, coffee, etc., since these may contain caffeine that will encourage you to urinate more. The alcohol will have the same effect, and so you will slowly lose fluid over the course of a night.

As a consequence, you become more and more dehydrated and one sign of dehydration is a headache.

Sleep disorders

The 'right' amount of sleep is a fine balance, and varies from individual to individual. However, we know that too much or too little sleep can be very damaging to health. Most people sleep around seven or eight hours each day, but the pattern of sleep often changes as people get older. Most people find it unavoidable now and then to 'undersleep', perhaps because of an early start to catch a holiday flight or because of occasional shift work. However, when people regularly sleep too much or too little they often experience a headache on waking, which at times can be quite persistent.

The first thing to rule out in a situation such as this is depression. Depression can contribute to headaches, and unusual sleeping patterns are also a sign of depression, especially oversleeping. If you generally feel very low and unhappy and are sleeping too much and, perhaps, spending less and less time with other people, you should consult your doctor.

Sleep apnoea is a disorder where breathing can stop when a person is sleeping. The person often wakes up many times during the night and can feel very tired in the morning. Essentially, the person experiences oxygen starvation during the night, often without being aware of it. If you often wake up feeling excessively tired and have headaches, this is a small possibility.

Another sleep-related cause is nocturnal tooth-grinding and jaw-clenching. If you grind your teeth together in your sleep, you not only wear your teeth down but you also overuse the jaw muscles, which can lead to headache during the day. If you sleep with a partner, he or she will often tell you about tooth grinding. Your dentist will also see signs of this and should tell you. If your dentist does not mention it, but you suspect it, ask him or her about it.

Stress

Stress probably affects all human beings, at least to some extent. In some societies it is caused by interpersonal conflict (arguments and disagreements, for instance) and by work; in others it may even be caused by fear for one's life (in dangerous political situations or in places where people are at risk from life-threatening events). In everyday life, even minor hassles, as they are called, contribute to stress. Queuing at the bank or waiting for a late train, having minor disputes with our neighbours, needing minor repairs to our cars and being served the wrong dish in a restaurant are all examples of little stressors that can add up for us. Stress is linked with anxiety and worry, and all contribute to headaches. Tension-type headaches are often called 'stress headaches' because they are often caused by muscle tension in the neck. We tend to tense up when stressed, hence the therapeutic value of a massage to relax us.

Health psychologists have spent many years studying stress because it can damage the body and the mind significantly and is so common. If you like, stress is to a health psychologist what cancer or heart disease is to a medical doctor. In the long term, stress can have a suppressant effect on the immune system. In fact, a branch of health psychology called psychoneuroimmunology is dedicated to this kind of effect. Therefore, a stressed person is much more likely to become ill, especially with viral infections such as colds and influenza. Of course, this is how a cycle can become established: stress causes illness, illness causes stress, and so on.

Identifying sources of stress in your life and trying to reduce stress by meditation, relaxation, or some other method, will certainly do you no harm and will almost definitely do you some good. If you suspect that your headaches are due to stress, or are made worse by stress, you should make an attempt to relax more. If you are overworking, you are probably stressing yourself and should perhaps try to step back a little and cut down on the hours that you spend working as opposed to relaxing and enjoying yourself. Your health *is* more important than work, even if at times it does not seem so.

HELPFUL TIPS! HELPFUL TIPS! HELPFUL TIPS! HELPFUL

One word of caution: if you resort to misusing alcohol or other drugs in order to relax you will store up other problems for yourself. Try to find other ways to de-stress.

Box 4. Research in brief: weekend headaches.

Psychologists and doctors are particularly interested in something called the 'weekend headache'. This is a headache which, unsurprisingly, occurs at the weekend. People look forward to the weekend to have a rest from work, and it can be very upsetting to find that most of that time is spent suffering from a headache. Why does this happen?

Torelli, Cologno and Manzoni (1999) investigated weekend headache, looking for lifestyle and work factors to explain this phenomenon. They compared a group of 31 weekend-headache patients with 19 other people who had different kinds of headache. The idea was that these two groups might differ in their lifestyles and work habits. They filled in a diary over a period of eight weeks to enable the researchers to identify particular patterns in their headache attacks. The researchers found that the weekend headache sufferers were having headaches at other times during the week, but the pattern of their work, and their leisure activities were such that they were more likely to judge their weekend headaches as feeling worse and being more painful or upsetting. This tells us that when people behave in certain ways, their headaches seem to react accordingly, and the people then react to their headaches. First, they might have work habits that lead to 'loose ends' for them to worry about every weekend, rather than leaving work each Friday knowing that everything is done. Work never leaves them, and so they have additional anxiety. They might invest a lot of effort in wanting to have a relaxed and fun weekend. The problem with this is that being desperate for something to happen can create a special kind of anxiety all of its own, and this can be stressful. This can then lead to headaches. When this starts to happen as a pattern, the person begins to worry at the end of each week that another headache will occur in the coming weekend. Of course, worrying about pain can induce the pain. Finally, the researchers discovered that an increased incidence of headaches at the weekend was only found in men. This suggests that there is something about the way men conduct and react to their work that brings on weekend headaches.

Eye strain

If you need spectacles and do not have them, or have them but they are no longer right for you, you may experience headaches. These can be caused by strain on the muscles in the eyes as they try to make the world clearer to you but are ill-equipped to do so. However, this can also be related to strain in the muscles in the face and head. Think of a person who is straining to see something; the strain shows on his or her face. If someone does this regularly over a period of days, weeks, months, and in many cases years, the strain placed on the muscles may lead to chronic headaches. The pain can obviously be in the eyes, but may be felt in the temples or forehead. You should have your eyes checked regularly to avoid this possibility.

HELPFUL TIPS! HELPFUL TIPS! HELPFUL TIPS! HELPFUL

Most opticians recommend eye-testing every two years, but if you notice that your vision seems to have changed then always see an optician, even if your eyes were tested only a week earlier.

Most people have 'floaters' in their field of vision. Floaters (also called *mouches volontes*) are dark specks that float across our view, and are especially noticeable when we are looking at a bright sky, or a whitewashed wall, or perhaps when reading a book. While many people never notice them, for some they can be an occasional distraction and for others a constant irritation. If you are aware of your floaters most of the time, then flicking the eyes around to watch them move, or trying to focus on them, can create eye strain and thus encourage headaches. There are no cures for floaters, unfortunately. However, if they are really making your life difficult then tinted lenses might help to tone down the environment and make them less noticeable. Speak to your optician, who will be able to see your floaters by examining the back of your eye.

Medication misuse

Medication misuse headache is becoming increasingly recognised by doctors, and is a rather ironic type of headache since it occurs because people are taking medication for headaches! We must not forget that all drugs are poisonous and, as such, have the capacity to cause problems. If you are taking medication regularly because of headaches, this medication itself can eventually create more and more headaches. If often occurs in people who are taking drugs for their migraines, where they may start to experience other headaches, often every day or every other day, between migraine attacks. When the medication is stopped, the person commonly stops having these daily headaches, and reverts back to having migraines at a frequency similar to what had occurred before he or she was prescribed drugs by the doctor. Obviously, no doctor wants to make your life worse with painkillers, and so if you seem to notice a pattern similar to this, please let your doctor know. The doctor will then usually stop your medication, and try other therapies, drugs or dosages until the best treatment for you is found.

Another thing to consider is that some kinds of painkillers can be quite addictive. If you are taking one regularly, then after a while you might need to stop taking that drug. One common withdrawal symptom is headache. Therefore, after a few hours or days of not using the drug, a headache may develop. Of course, taking a different painkiller stops the headache, but for the wrong reasons. If you have been taking certain painkillers regularly for a long time, especially those containing drugs such as codeine, speak to your doctor about any concerns you might have.

Hypertension

People with high blood pressure often experience headaches. In fact, it can be one of the only signs that you have hypertension. All persistent headaches should be checked out with your doctor, and your doctor should test your blood pressure if you ask him or her about your headaches.

Most people have experienced episodes of what is called *postural hyper-tension*. This is, basically, temporarily increased pressure to the head when a person bends down. It may be accompanied by visual disturbance in the form of flashing lights in the field of vision. Usually the hypertension is relieved when the posture changes again. For persons who are prone to this condition, headaches may be a consequence of the episode. However, if this happens to you regularly, you should speak to your doctor.

Dental problems

Dental problems are common, and can be the cause of certain headaches. Caries or 'holes' in teeth are what the dentist fills with a 'plug', which is either mercury-based or made from some other material such as a form of plastic or porcelain. Abscesses can form at the roots of infected teeth, and even cause nerve damage. Some teeth do not grow properly and impact on each other. All of these cause pain. Most of the time we know the difference between a pain in the tooth and a pain in the head, but not always. There is something called 'referred pain', which is where a problem in one place causes a pain in another.

A very rare cause of chronic headaches, disputed by some, can be mercury poisoning. Every time you bite down on a mercury filling, a tiny amount of mercury is emitted, which can be breathed in. All ingested mercury does not leave the body once it enters. Some remains there forever, and over time can build up. In certain individuals who are particularly sensitive to mercury, headaches can result. If you have mercury fillings in almost every tooth of your mouth (something not uncommon in older individuals who eat sugary foods and do not take care of their teeth), then the chances of this problem increase. This is, as mentioned earlier, very rare, and should only be investigated where all other possibilities have been exhausted. It should be pointed out that, in the UK, mercury poisoning from dental fillings is not considered, by official bodies, to be a health risk.

HELPFUL TIPS! HELPFUL TIPS! HELPFUL TIPS! HELPFUL

Remember that headaches can also be caused by problems with the teeth, and you should therefore visit your dentist regularly.

Ear infection

Pain in the ear can also be mistaken for headache. Ear pain usually occurs because of infection, which is relatively easy to cure with antibiotics or other readily available treatments. In certain cases, a doctor might refer a patient with headaches to an otorhinolaryngologist, or ear, nose and throat (ENT) specialist. Again, this is another good reason why you should see your doctor if you have persistent headaches.

Sinusitis

This is an infection in the cavities of the bone in the nose and forehead. Because of where it is, it creates pain similar to a headache, and can be confused for migraine and vice versa. A person with sinusitis is likely to have other symptoms, such as sneezing, dripping nose, redness and tenderness in the upper face, and possibly a fever. The pain should be worse if the head is lowered, for instance when bending down to pick something up. Sinusitis is best treated by antibiotics, but this, unfortunately, will not reduce the effect of migraines.

Exertion

You can induce a headache by straining your body. This can be quite normal, and is only a problem if it occurs often, or if the headache you experience is genuinely intense, or if it is accompanied by other symptoms such as flashes of light, blurring of vision, unusual tastes and so on. Sneezing, coughing, lifting heavy weights and so on all put strain on the body and increase the pressure in the head – hence the headache. Sometimes, it is necessary to exert yourself when on the toilet, and this too puts additional pressure on the blood vessels in the head. While you cannot avoid sneezing and coughing, you can certainly take more care when exercising or lifting, and if it is difficult to pass a stool, it may be advisable to wait until you are ready to do so naturally, or to use a laxative in moderation. Persistent constipation, however, is best reported to your doctor. Problems with passing stools are often the result of poor diet, and your doctor can help you to identify ways in which you can change your diet to make your digestive system (and hence your whole body) healthier.

Anxiety

Worry creates stress, and stress creates headaches. Furthermore, worrying about headaches that you experience can generate more and worse headaches. This is why you should see your doctor rather than dwell upon headaches and wonder about their causes. The mere fact that you are reading this book shows that you have already taken some positive steps towards sorting out the problem. Hopefully, this will help to reduce any anxiety you are experiencing.

Noise pollution

If you have ever been to a pop concert and been too-close-for-comfort to the speakers, you may have left with a ringing in your ears and a headache. Noise can generate a headache and can come from a number of sources. Perhaps your car stereo is too loud? Perhaps you work with noisy machines or live near a very busy road? Are your children excessively noisy? Do you live with someone who talks very loudly? All in all, some of these may sound silly but could lead to headaches in the short or long term. While you may have difficulty telling your partner to be less noisy, you certainly can ask your employer for ear protection if you work with machinery and usually this will be expected to be provided, by law.

Light pollution

Any form of light can be the cause of a headache. Even natural sunlight may trigger pain if you immerse yourself in it too much. However, non-natural light is a more common cause that has been identified. This comes from two main sources: television and computer screens, and fluorescent lighting. Watching a lot of television, playing computer games excessively, and being exposed to artificial lights, either at home or at work or in the form of neon lights in cities, all may contribute to light pollution headaches or migraines. Furthermore, it is very common for people at work to be using computers most of the day while sitting under fluorescent strip lights. The potential for a problem is therefore greater in these circumstances. In no circumstances should you use a fluorescent light when it starts to flicker. Investigate the problem immediately and correct it, or simply do not use the light. If a light at work flickers, report it immediately. Flickering lights are even more of a problem, because they can trigger an epileptic seizure even in people who are not diagnosed as epileptic. It is relatively rare, but possible.

Neuralgia

This is pain generated from a particular nerve in the face; it is not strictly a headache, although some people may think it is. Others may confuse it for toothache. It is very strong and often occurs in response to a trigger such as wind on the face or putting your head on a pillow. People with neuralgia usually experience a 'lightning strike' of pain down one side of the face, mainly over the cheek. It can also be mistaken for a cluster headache.

Rarer causes

Altitude changes

One could argue that this is a rare cause for most readers of this book, since the majority will not live in mountainous areas or regularly travel up and down. However, a lot of people on earth do this, and tourists and sports figures also experience altitude sickness. Most people will be aware of some of the aspects of this, but may not be aware of the intense headache or migraine that can be brought on by changes in altitude. The following account best demonstrates what can happen.

> **❝**I experienced altitude sickness, in the form of severe headache, in the Peruvian Andes. Having never been at high altitude before, so having no idea whether or not I would be affected by altitude sickness, or in what way, I had taken recommended precautions to avoid it, such as drinking large amounts of water, sucking glucose sweets, and avoiding alcohol.

However, the best method of avoiding it is considered to be gradual acclimatisation; in other words, ascending slowly over a number of days. Unfortunately, I did not have the opportunity to do this.

On reaching 4800m, I experienced only slight dizziness, to be expected on account of the lack of oxygen, and confidently believed that I was not going to suffer any altitude sickness. But, during the afternoon, shortly after reaching the town, I noticed that I had started to develop a nagging headache. This got progressively worse during the afternoon and evening. I was advised to take whatever I would usually take for a headache, so took ibuprofen, but this seemed to have no effect on the pain. During dinner that evening my head was pounding to the point where I felt sick. My head also felt extremely tender, and it was uncomfortable to move it, or to walk, since it throbbed with each step. I went to bed very early, in the hope that it would be gone in the morning.

When I woke up the pain was considerably worse. I was unable to move my head, even slightly on the pillow, without sharp, stabbing pain, followed by prolonged throbbing. My whole head felt as if it was bruised and something was pressing on the bruising. Light, both natural and artificial, was extremely painful and I could not tolerate it for any length of time; in addition I was, most alarmingly, experiencing some visual disturbance, with objects appearing to be slightly distorted, seeming either convex or concave. Painkillers were still having no noticeable effect. I managed to get up, slowly and painfully, but was unable to eat breakfast, since actions like chewing and swallowing hurt my head, and I found it difficult to talk to anyone, since even this amount of movement could set the stabbing off again.

The most worrying aspect was trying to determine exactly how bad this needed to get before there was cause for serious concern. I knew that with mild altitude sickness, known as soroche, the symptoms should die down reasonably quickly, but that if they did not go, or if they became worse, I would need to go down to a lower altitude as quickly as possible. However, I had no idea how severe a pain could be within 'normal' limits, or just how quickly I should expect it to go away.

On getting on the tour bus, I tried to go to sleep as soon as possible, but this was somewhat difficult on account of the discomfort caused by the bus rattling along unpaved, pot-holed, roads. I felt as if my brain was rattling around inside my skull. On stopping for a break, I was unable to get off the bus, or even to open my eyes on account of the bright light.

The Peruvian guide and bus driver were concerned by this time, and suggested that I tried chewing coca leaves, as the locals do to combat soroche. They gave me a small parcel of the leaves, wrapped around a tiny block of resin, to put inside my cheek and chew periodically. This tasted bitter and was thoroughly unpleasant, but, to my surprise, it did indeed lessen the pain. Although it did not alleviate it completely, it certainly seemed to take the edge off the sharpness of the stabbing, and I seemed to be able to see more clearly and to bear the light better.

I chewed the leaves on and off all day while travelling. While I cannot say that the headache would not have receded by itself, I did feel that this had made a considerable difference. That night, I was back down to 2300m, and, after a few hours at this level, the pain disappeared completely. Fortunately, it did not come back again during my time in the Andes, even when I returned to high altitude. However, I did carry coca leaves with me after that, just in case.**"**

Amelia, 33

The important thing to do is to take care and follow appropriate advice. If you are going to suffer altitude sickness, there is probably no way of completely avoiding it, but being careful can certainly reduce the suffering that is likely to occur. If you are a migraineur, please be aware that there is a very good chance that travelling at high altitudes could trigger an attack. Although you might want to see the world, there are certain places that might be out of bounds for you for health reasons.

Nutritional causes

Basically, just about anything you eat or drink, or what you do not eat or drink, can lead to a headache. However, these causes are listed with the rarer ones because they are often undiagnosed, and so cases of diagnosed food-related headaches are not common. Food is made up of chemicals, like in fact everything in the world, including you. Sometimes people react badly to those chemicals and sometimes they are allergic to them. Reacting badly and being allergic are not the same things, but it is not necessary to explain the subtleties of the differences here. Suffice it to say that allergies are an immune reaction, whereas a sensitivity to something might not be an allergy. Chinese people can react quite badly to alcohol, and can often be very ill and drunk on just small quantities. This, however, is because of their body chemistry and is not an allergy.

Two of the most common headache-causing foods are chocolate and cheese. Cheese contains a substance known as *tyramine*, which is believed to be the reason for its headache-producing qualities. It is a chemical that acts upon blood vessels, causing them to change in diameter, which we know is directly related to migraine specifically. If you suspect that cheese may be responsible for your migraines, try cottage cheese instead, which does not contain tyramine.

The tyramine present in cheese belongs to a family of chemicals known as *amines*. These are quite natural substances that are present in most things, but some people can be particularly sensitive to them, especially in larger doses. Chocolate contains a number of amines. However, although chocolate can be a trigger for migraines, it can also be a scapegoat for other, less easily identifiable causes. As a psychologist, I am only too aware that often what people perceive is quite different from the reality of a situation. It is, therefore, quite easy to blame chocolate for your migraines. Just before a migraine, people commonly crave sugar because the blood-sugar levels in the body are lower than usual. Of course, chocolate is a common source of sugar, so it is the first port of call. Then the migraine takes effect, and people quite logically assume that the chocolate caused the migraine. Actually, in such cases it is more likely to be what we would call a 'coincident factor'. Let us take a slightly more obvious example: if you noticed that every time it rained you had sore feet, you might think that the rain was causing the soreness. However, people would not jump to this conclusion. They might simply work out that in the rain they wore a particular pair of shoes which they did not wear at any other time. Therefore, the shoes cause the soreness, but the rain triggers the wearing of the shoes.

Now we can return to another source of confusion, related to the first issue. Women may experience migraines related to their menstrual cycle. As you may be aware, craving sugary foods like chocolate is very common when women are premenstrual and again this is related to low blood-sugar levels. It is possible then for a premenstrual woman to identify the chocolate as a cause of her migraine, when actually it is really related to her period.

Caffeine is another potential trigger for headaches and migraines. It is possible to consume a large amount of caffeine because it is present in such common foodstuffs as tea, coffee, cola drinks and chocolate. If you drink tea or coffee throughout the day, have one or two caffeine-rich soft drinks, and eat chocolate for your dessert, you may be overdosing on caffeine. Apart from headaches, you may experience problems with your digestive system. The best thing to do is to avoid these things altogether. Some people may recommend switching to decaffeinated drinks, but this does not solve the problem completely. Caffeine is only one of a family of substances that are present in coffee, etc. When the manufacturers remove the caffeine, the 'cousins' of caffeine are still present and they, too, can have the same action. However, these 'cousins' are weaker, and if your headaches are caused by these chemicals you are likely to notice a reduction in symptoms by switching to decaffeinated drinks – even if the problem is not eradicated completely.

Note, however, that withdrawal from caffeine and its 'cousins' can cause headaches and migraines. They are quite powerful drugs, even though you might not realise it, and there is a period of 'cold turkey' associated with withdrawal. You may feel more irritable and therefore stressed, which again may trigger headaches. You may feel more tired than usual, because caffeine is a stimulant – it jogs the system, keeping you alert and awake. Be careful that you do not sleep too much if you reduce your intake of caffeine, because the additional sleep can also cause headaches.

Just as eating certain substances can be responsible for migraines, it is also important to be aware that lack of food can also be a cause. If you do not eat regularly, or if you sometimes spend long periods of time without eating (such as during religious fastings), you may create migraines by artificially lowering your blood-sugar level. If you seem to be experiencing migraines associated with fasting in particular, speak to your local religious leader. He is likely to allow you to opt out of the tradition on health grounds, or at least to make a token gesture towards fasting without engaging with it wholly.

HELPFUL TIPS! HELPFUL TIPS! HELPFUL TIPS! HELPFUL

- If you suspect that chocolate is causing a migraine, try switching to another sugary substance, such as boiled sweets. If the migraines still occur, then it is not chocolate *per se* that is to blame, but something else and you should see your doctor.

- You should cut down on caffeine before you cut it out. Caffeine is a stimulant. Allow your body (and mind) time to adjust.

Diabetes

Headaches can result from diabetes, because diabetes is often associated with high blood pressure. Of course, as we have seen elsewhere, hypertension can be associated with headaches. However, when migraineurs develop diabetes they often report that their migraines are less severe. This is likely to be due to changes in blood-sugar levels. People who gain weight often have relief from migraines, and again this may be due to increases in blood sugar, since the reason that people gain weight is usually that they are eating more. Eating more leads to higher levels of blood sugar. As you can see, it is a complicated system!

When people with diabetes have migraines, it is often found that the migraines are at their worst when the diabetes is badly controlled. If diabetes affects you it is important that you take the advice of your doctor and stick to the medication and lifestyle that has been recommended.

Thyrotoxicosis

When people have an overactive thyroid they can experience an increase in migraines. As with diabetes, controlling the thyroid function can help with the migraines, and so be aware that if you have been diagnosed with an overactive thyroid you should mention any migraines you have had to the doctor.

Temporal arteritis (giant cell arteritis)

This is a relatively common cause of headaches, but only in people over the age of 60. We do not yet know why it happens and it can be confused with tension-type headache. In temporal arteritis, the arteries in the temples tend to be noticeable to the eye, and are tender to the touch. There is often a throbbing pain over the eye and temple, but pain can also be felt in the neck or back of the head. Often, soreness of the scalp is found; there is sometimes pain when chewing; and weight loss may occur. Most people can be cured of this problem by using steroidal drugs, although a small number of people do not respond to treatment. The majority of patients must take the drugs permanently and the consequences of not receiving treatment for temporal arteritis are serious. Blindness is one likely outcome, and it could occur suddenly. However, it must be stressed that the success rate of treatment is quite high.

Rare causes

When people experience headaches, especially those that cannot easily be softened by painkillers, they often worry that they are experiencing the symptoms of a brain tumour or a stroke or something similarly dramatic. While headaches *are* symptomatic of a tumour in the brain, tumours are very rarely the cause, and you should bear this in mind while reading this section.

Carbon monoxide poisoning

Gas-powered appliances (heating systems and ovens) in your home or workplace release carbon monoxide, a very toxic but odourless substance. Regular exposure to high levels of carbon monoxide will kill. Normally, the flue for such appliances deals with carbon monoxide, but this does not always occur, and high levels of carbon monoxide can be released from malfunctioning cookers, fires and boilers. If you are exposed to high levels of carbon monoxide, you are likely to have persistent headaches and sleepiness, and aching in the body, similar to the symptoms of influenza. To avoid this you should have your appliances checked regularly, and fit carbon monoxide detectors in your home.

Lead and mercury poisoning

Both of these 'heavy metals', as they are referred to by chemists, are highly toxic and tend to build up in the body. We all have trace quantities of lead and mercury in our bodies, but if people are regularly exposed to these substances they can start to feel very ill indeed and eventually people subjected to enough lead or mercury will die.

If you work with either or both of these substances you will almost certainly be well protected, since this is legally required. However, if you have any doubts then these should be investigated. If you do not work with lead or mercury then you are extremely unlikely to have headaches linked to them. Bear in mind, however, that some old metal models are made from lead, and many older paints contained lead. While modern paints are much safer in this respect, you should remember that your house might have been painted in the past using lead-based paints. So, ensure that your children do not eat scraps of dried paint that may be flaking from windowsills, doors, etc.

HELPFUL TIPS! HELPFUL TIPS! HELPFUL TIPS! HELPFUL

Take precautions when stripping or sanding down old paints, since the dust you are creating could be highly toxic.

Bacterial and viral infection

Meningitis can be caused by both bacterial and viral infection, but it is the bacterial form that is more harmful. In the worst cases it progresses extremely rapidly and causes death. However, this is not what usually happens, and there is a very good recovery rate. Meningitis is very rare, but there are 'outbreaks' at certain times which can cause concern, especially when they are sensationalised in the press. The symptoms include headaches, but also a fever, neck stiffness, vomiting, hypersensitivity to light and a rash of pink or purple blemishes which do not recede when pressure is applied to them. Meningitis usually affects children and younger people, but can affect anyone. Again, it is extremely rare, but if you do know someone who starts to have a fever, stiff neck, headaches, a rash, nausea and cannot bear light (or a smaller set of these symptoms) then contact a doctor immediately. Please bear in mind, however, that migraines themselves can also be associated with photophobia (dislike of light). If you have *only* a strong headache and a desire to sit in the dark, you are almost certainly experiencing a migraine rather than signs of meningitis.

Benign tumours

These are essentially lumps of tissue in the brain which will not spread. Because they are not likely to grow, in many ways the worst has already happened. Surgery can be performed to remove the tumour, since it is a distinct object that can be found within the brain. Sometimes, the tumour can be left where it is, if the doctors are satisfied that it is not causing any significant problems for the patient. The signs and symptoms are similar to those listed below for malignant tumours.

Malignant tumours

These are also lumps in the brain, but this time they are likely to grow and spread. They are what most people call cancer, although strictly speaking benign tumours are also a form of cancer. The cells proliferate, and spread into other cells. In extreme cases they travel to other parts of the body and continue to spread there. The first thing to be aware of is that survival rates are not high in this particular case. However, your headache is unlikely to be due to a brain tumour. If you *only* experience headaches, then you are *extremely* unlikely to have this problem. Most patients with brain tumours go to their doctor because of one or more of the other symptoms. These include blindness, other visual disturbances, numbness or paralysis, slurring of speech or forgetting of words, vomiting, fainting, or altered perceptions of reality. Headache is rarely the only symptom. Even if you have some of the other symptoms, you could simply have migraine. After all, migraines can also affect vision and speech, can cause digestive disturbance and can even generate hallucinations. Therefore, do not think the worst when reading this section. Furthermore, the majority of people who develop malignant brain tumours are either children or the elderly. You might be in the lowest risk group of all.

If you are concerned about working out the difference between the symptoms of a brain tumour and those of a migraine, you should bear in mind the following things. First, headaches are usually only a later symptom of a brain tumour, after some of the other symptoms listed above have occurred. Second, with migraine, things such as speech problems or visual disturbance occur in the same timeframe as the headache. In the case of a brain tumour, a person may experience a visual disturbance entirely on its own, or vomit for no apparent reason. Again, please remember that people do vomit for lots of reasons, and the vast majority of these are in no way connected with brain tumours.

In the rare cases of malignant brain tumours, doctors may perform surgery if the tumour is at an early stage and has not spread. When the cancer has spread (a process known as *metastasis*), radiotherapy and chemotherapy are the probable treatments.

Trauma and bleeding

First, the term *trauma* should be explained. To the average person this means 'something awful that happens'. Doctors use the term differently, to mean a physical accident that occurs. If you bump your head, or stub your toe, these are examples of trauma. If you cut off your finger while slicing bread, this is also trauma. It is basically the medical word for 'injury'. (Doctors also use the term for psychological injury.) Head injuries are quite common, but serious head injuries are less so. Most of us have hurt our head climbing into or out of a car, or something similar, and we may even have had a headache afterwards. That is to be expected, but if a headache is particularly strong or has unusual symptoms, or lasts more than a day, the advice of a doctor should be sought. If a blow to the head has caused a person to lose consciousness, he or she should always be taken to a doctor. Most of the time, all will be fine, but it must be investigated.

A blow to the head does not carry with it any serious issues *per se*. The problem is that further injuries may arise as a result. The skull may fracture or break. If it does, it may cause internal bleeding, or produce pressure in the head. Pressure and bleeding in the head should be investigated immediately as both may cause lasting damage to the brain. In the short term they are likely to create headaches, but are usually associated with other neurological symptoms such as flashes of light, blurred or double vision, dizziness, nausea, vomiting, numbness, speech problems and so on. It is also possible for bleeding to occur in the head without any damage to the external bone, which is why any significant blow to the head, accompanied by persistent headache, should be investigated.

Bleeding is referred to by doctors as a haemorrhage, and there are many reasons for this to occur. Some people have high blood pressure, matched with thin or weak points in the blood vessels. Of course, high pressure in a weak vessel can mean that the vessel bursts, and this is what happens in the case of sub-arachnoid haemorrhage. This is something that becomes more common as we age but is still relatively rare. In the most extreme case the person would have a very sudden and extremely painful headache. It would feel as if he or she had been hit with a cannonball. A stiff neck would be another sign that would come on very quickly, and the person may even lose consciousness. The later consequences would be similar to those of a stroke; the person may be unable to speak, may have paralysis, and so on.

Of course, any accident can cause some bleeding in the head, even in perfectly healthy people with no evidence of weakness in the cardiovascular system. This is why all major and unusual accidents must be investigated by a doctor.

Headaches of unidentifiable origin

Sometimes, a doctor simply cannot find the reason for a patient's headaches. This might be because all the possibilities have not been explored, but it will more likely be that such headaches are predominantly psychological. Realistically, your doctor is only likely to check out the *probable* causes of your problem, not every single one of them. Be prepared for your doctor to stop looking once he or she has ruled out all of the dangerous or life-threatening problems. After that, you may be on your own. For many people – especially when the headaches or migraines are truly psychological – a visit to the doctor usually gives them significant relief from the problem, and sometimes permanently.

Remember that there are thousands of possible causes of headaches. This book can only deal with a small proportion of them, and the vast majority of headaches are quite harmless. However, it is always sensible to check out any unusual symptoms or persistent or strong headaches.

Points to note

- There are hundreds of causes of migraines and headaches. You name it, and it probably triggers an attack in someone.
- Most headaches are *not* signs of a dangerous or serious medical problem.
- Always check out strong, persistent headaches with your doctor.

What are the consequences?

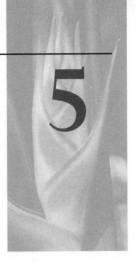

The consequences of medical conditions are almost always mainly psychological. You *think* and *feel* things about your illness, and your illness can affect what you think and feel.

The consequences of headache and migraine vary greatly from person to person. What is unbearable to one person can be tolerable to another. However, one thing is very important: if you are suffering from headaches or migraines, do not just tolerate them. You really should seek help and treatment. If you do not, the consequences could be serious. Headaches can make you irritable, depressed or, in the worse cases, suicidal. To avoid the long-term effects of headaches, try to find some remedy. Even if you do not succeed in curing them, just knowing that you have tried to stop them can be comforting, because you feel as if you have made an effort. If you give in to them, it will often make you feel worse and helpless. Most people, if they try, can help themselves in a variety of health complaints, and taking control of your health is never a bad thing.

What follows is all about psychology, rather than medicine.

The short term

During or immediately after a headache or migraine there are some things you should think about. The most important is that you should not operate machinery or drive with anything other than a mild headache. This may come as a shock to some of you, who, if necessary, will drive with a strong headache, but you really should not. The main reason is simply that pain is distracting. When in pain, you concentrate on the pain more than on other things, which is potentially dangerous when driving or using machinery. Of course, it is also true that other things can distract you from pain, and this is why driving might actually take your mind off your headache when the headache is only mild. When the pain is stronger, however, and you find that you need to concentrate on it in order to deal with it, you will not be able to use all of your attention to avoid getting involved in accidents on the road or in the workplace. As psychologists know, people are not always aware that they are concentrating less, just as drivers under the influence of even a small amount of alcohol are not always aware that their senses are impaired. Psychologists talk of things such as 'feeling of knowing' and 'self-awareness'. Normally, you do not only do things, or say things, but you know you are doing them and saying them. There may be times, however, when you don't. Have you ever seen a person delirious with fever, who is saying things without knowing it? Have you ever talked while asleep? We monitor ourselves all of the time, in a kind of feedback loop. One of the reasons that we cannot walk around easily with a blindfold is because the loop has been broken. We are not getting the information from our eyes that allows us to adjust our movements. Now, when we are distracted by something, these processes of monitoring are among the first to suffer. We are still able to do things, but we suffer in our ability to be aware of what we are doing. This is why we can put our spectacles somewhere and then have to hunt for them because we have forgotten where we put them. We *did* put them somewhere; we did carry out the physical act. We simply acted in a kind of automatic mode, perhaps because our mind was on something else. As you can see, if our minds are partly used up thinking about our pain, we will have less concentration available to us.

This problem runs deeper as migraines, in particular, can affect your senses. You might fail to see things that are there, or see shapes and colours that are not. Imagine the situation, when driving, where you swerve to avoid something you *think* is there, but collide with something you had not noticed.

Box 5.	Research in brief: effects on concentration.

The following research supports the case that we are not able to concentrate properly when we are having a headache or a migraine. Meyer et al. (2000) conducted a study of mental abilities in 199 people experiencing cluster headaches, migraines with and without aura, and some other types of headache. They tracked them over 10 years, regularly testing them at intervals of between 3 and 12 months. They gave them two tests, the Mini-Mental Status Examination and the Cognitive Capacity Screening Examination. Both tests involve asking ▶

people to do relatively simple tasks such as naming the President or Prime Minister, knowing what day it is, following instructions, and copying drawings. Regardless of the type of headache, people undergoing them showed significant decline in their thinking skills. When they were not having headaches, their scores went back up to normal. So, the good news is that the cognitive decline is reversible. The bad news is that you really should think twice about driving or operating machinery when you have a headache or migraine.

For those people who have stronger headaches or migraines the advice is simple. If you get a warning that you are going to get a headache or migraine, stop what you are doing and go home while you still can get there safely. If you get no warning, and you are in the throes of a strong headache or migraine, stop what you are doing and try to find a way to get home which does not involve driving. If you cannot get home, make suitable arrangements. It is not always practicable to act on this advice, but you should do so whenever you can.

One other issue needs to be raised. When you are in pain, your mood can change. You can become irritable, impatient, and so on. If you can avoid making really important decisions at these times, it is desirable. Furthermore, try to avoid getting into an argument with a friend, family member or colleague. The last thing you want is to say something in anger which you later regret or have to try to retract. In addition, arguments are likely to worsen your headache.

The long term

In the longer term, over months or years, having chronic headaches can affect the way you think about the world. They can also affect your behaviour. Any illness or condition over a protracted period of time can do this, and psychologists who study chronic illness are very aware of it.

Those who have had a condition for any length of time will tell you that they are really sick and tired of it. This is quite normal and natural. In the case of headaches and migraine, people often start to worry about the next occurrence. They are aware that the condition is 'hanging over them', ready to strike. So, after some time, people start to feel uneasy. As we also know, worrying about a headache can induce a headache, and this is particularly troublesome. Most people who suffer from headaches will say that they make them anxious and worried, and this is when long-term psychological factors can become problematic. Anxiety is something that psychologists take very seriously. Over the months and years, your levels of anxiety can increase, creating further problems. You can become more and more worried about your health and the worry creates stress. Stress can directly affect your health. It can cause skin conditions like eczema, or it can bring on headaches. A negative cycle is thus established, which can really only be broken by changing your views about things, and learning to relax – something with which a psychologist can help.

To avoid the stress–headache cycle, you must take steps to relax whenever you can, which will also help to reduce the frequency of your headaches.

Another important issue is that of 'social support'. This is a fancy term used by psychologists to describe the help we get in life from friends and family. Having a shoulder to cry on, or someone to baby-sit now and then so that we can have a night out, are important to us. Of course, headaches and migraines are very much a solitary activity. The more of them we

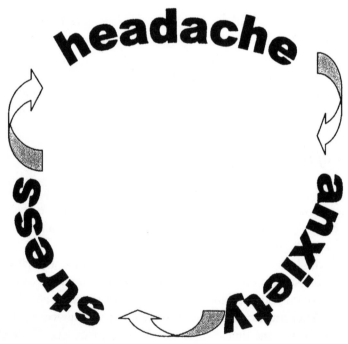

Stress–anxiety–headache cycle.

have, the more we spend time alone, in the quiet, perhaps in the dark, away from people because we need to avoid high levels of light and noise. If this keeps on happening over a longer period of time, it could affect our social relationships. If someone cannot go out with friends to a bar because the noise, the smoke, etc., bring on a migraine, then that person may see his or her friends less and less. Now, psychologists know that when people have high levels of social support they are better able to deal with illness and its effects. Therefore, any illness that can create some social isolation needs to be managed very carefully. The advice is to make sure that you do spend time with friends, no matter how common your headaches may be. If you cannot engage in the usual activities with friends, find some time to see them in other environments, perhaps going for a walk or visiting each others' homes. Do not allow your condition to affect your friendships or family relationships.

Gloomy times

Although it is not extremely common, some people can become depressed during the course of a chronic condition – and this can also affect headache and migraine sufferers. Day after day, week after week, year after year, a medical problem hanging over you, affecting many aspects of your normal life, begins to get you down. Depression is a frightening word to many people, although it does not necessarily mean that being depressed is always to be viewed as such a terrible thing. Many people have depression in the course of their life, and it is not always as debilitating as in the most extreme cases – although, of course, it is usually only the most extreme cases we hear about. Most depression, when it occurs, is manageable, and people do get 'cured'. Depression may occur, in headache and migraine sufferers, because of the long-term worry and stress caused by the condition and by a loss of social support. In cases where migraine is very frequent and very strong, people may have to give up their jobs, and this can be the sort of situation where depression can grow unless it is well managed. Remember that word: *managed*. Psychologists talk about managing health and illness, and this is very important because it tells us a crucial thing: you are the boss, not your illness. If you take control, you can win.

If, over time, you start to feel that you are losing energy, perhaps sleeping more, and caring less about things, then it is worth talking to your doctor. If you treat such problems early, they are more easily remedied, just like a physical illness.

Points to note

- The consequences of headaches and migraines vary from person to person.
- In the short term, avoid operating machinery or driving when having a headache or migraine.
- Do not make really important decisions or argue with someone when you are in strong pain. There is evidence that your judgement is temporarily affected.
- Chronic headaches can lead to long-term unhappiness. Try to seek help and do not suffer in silence.

What treatments are available?

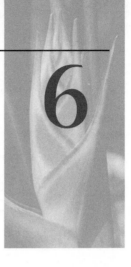

This chapter deals with the more common treatments, since these can make a big difference to the health of the majority of people experiencing headaches or migraines.

Medical and physical approaches

Most remedies for headaches and migraines are quite simple and have little or no side-effects. In fact, the most common remedies, such as drugs to kill pain, are widely available, even without prescription. In some cases, prescription drugs are necessary, and in a very small number of cases surgery may be necessary to remove some blockage or obstruction.

Orthodox medicine

The most obvious of orthodox medical therapies is that of analgesia. Indeed, the first response is usually to deal with the pain, and to consider the causes after that. There are a great many painkillers, varying in strength, method of action, and toxicity. The three main drugs widely available without prescription are aspirin, paracetamol and ibuprofen. In the short term these can be very effective, but if your headaches last more than a few days you should stop taking them and see your doctor. This is particularly important because your body can adjust to these drugs in such a way that over a period of time you can actually develop a headache when you stop taking them, just as you can develop a headache when you stop drinking tea or coffee if you normally drink these beverages daily.

Sometimes, especially when you are experiencing headaches due to some kind of allergic reaction – including such things as hay fever – your doctor may advise that you take antihistamines. These drugs suppress the immune system and stop your body reacting strongly to the allergen (in the case of hay fever, this is airborne pollen). Some antihistamines can make you sleepy, which of course means that you should not drive or operate machinery after taking them. Check your information leaflet carefully when you take a drug.

Box 6. **Research in brief: doctor–patient relationships.**

Psychologists are very aware of the gap that sometimes exists between doctor and patient. You probably don't share much with your doctor because his or her life could be quite different from yours, and his or her upbringing or culture could also be different. These things, and others, mean that when you try to talk to your doctor and your doctor talks to you there may be some loss of essential information. People often complain because their doctor does not explain things well, or because the doctor is too busy to listen to them. As psychologists, we are aware that this can have an impact on the success of your treatment, or on the way you follow the advice you have been given. Anne MacGregor (1997), in the journal *Neurology*, points out that, with respect to migraines, the doctor might have a slightly different agenda from the patient. Doctors are good at curing things, but not always so good at making patients feel better about things. She recommends that doctors should spend time listening to their migraine patients, understanding their triggers, and tailoring their care and treatment to their individual circumstances. Success of treatment can depend on these things. Using the recommendations from MacGregor's advice to doctors, we can generate a list of things you can expect and ask your doctor to do. They are:

- That your doctor should listen to your expertise about your own headaches.
- That your doctor should identify any triggers that you have noticed.
- That all advice should be clearly explained, and that your doctor should ask to make sure you do grasp what is being said.
- That your doctor should explain any treatments being offered and explain in simple terms why they work.
- That your doctor should want to see you at regular intervals during the course of your treatment to follow up the result of what has been suggested.

Complementary therapies

A wide range of complementary therapies are available which, it is claimed, ameliorate headaches and migraine. When reading about these, please bear in mind that they are intended to *complement* orthodox medicine, not to replace it. This is why we no longer tend to use the term 'alternative medicine'. If you decide to take advantage of what complementary therapies have to offer, make sure that you have also sought advice from your doctor about your headaches. After all, *the vast majority of complementary practitioners are not medically qualified.* Complementary therapies can, for some people, make a big difference, but there are some things they simply cannot do. If you are having headaches because of a perforated ear drum, for example, no amount of reflexology or homeopathy will alter such a clearly physical ailment. In fact, sometimes complementary therapies can be a problem because they may deal with the pain, making you think that the problem has gone away, but the underlying cause may still be there. Therefore, do the right thing and see your doctor in addition to any other therapies you seek.

Acupuncture

More and more doctors are willing to prescribe acupuncture to their patients, and there is some evidence to suggest that it can work much beyond the placebo effect. It is a part of Chinese medicine, but can be used as a stand-alone treatment. It involves the insertion of very fine needles into the skin, to a depth of around three to six millimetres. A herb may also be burned around the area – a process known as *moxibustion.* Many people worry that acupuncture will be painful, and for some people it is, although the amount of pain experienced is often small and most patients would say that this is a small price to pay for the benefits they receive. There are university courses to train people in acupuncture, and it is generally taken seriously as a therapeutic approach, although it still has its opponents. If you are squeamish about needles, there is a friendly alternative in the form of *acupressure.* This is based upon the same philosophy as acupuncture but involves massage of certain points on the body rather than the insertion of needles.

If you can get access to acupuncture or acupressure just before a migraine strikes, you are quite likely to experience some relief, and perhaps may avoid the attack altogether. However, this is a difficult thing to do, of course, as there are no 'emergency acupuncturists' waiting on call. Non-emergency courses of acupuncture have been shown to work for some people, but do not necessarily give permanent relief.

Feverfew and other herbs and plants

Feverfew (*Tanacetum parthenium*) is a natural remedy that some people have used to relieve their migraines. It is a member of the sunflower family, and its leaves were used by the Ancient Greeks not only as a remedy for migraine, but also as an anti-inflammatory drug for conditions such as arthritis. It works against the action of serotonin, a substance which, as mentioned earlier, is involved in migraine. It is generally safe for most people to take, although it can create stomach upset. Migraines and joint pains can occur if people stop taking it – a type of withdrawal effect. Some research suggests that it can be effective, although there is still quite a debate as to its usefulness. As with most complementary medicines, it works for some people. It does not matter why it works, as long as it does and provided that it will not injure health. Therefore, you might try it for your headaches, but be aware that you should not stop taking it suddenly, but in stages, otherwise the withdrawal effects above might occur.

There are other herbs and plant extracts that can help your headache or migraine. If you are interested in these, it is best to do some reading, but remember that you could be swamped with advice from websites, books and therapists. In the end, you should make your own choice as to what you try, preferably in consultation with your doctor, since the chemicals in some plants can be harmful if taken when you have high blood pressure, or are pregnant, or are taking certain other drugs, and so on. To give you an idea of how big a market there is for herbal remedies for headaches and migraine, here is a list of a small fraction of the plants that some people claim will make a difference: cayenne pepper, meadowsweet, peppermint, rosemary, kava, neem, peony, marijuana, cotton, echinacea, foxglove, primrose, basil, passion flower, sage, wintergreen, marjoram, betony, tansy and thyme.

One more word of advice: do not try more than one possible remedy at the same time. When scientists (whether psychologists or chemists or doctors) want to investigate the effects of a drug or some other treatment, they do things systematically. They test out one remedy at a time, giving a period of 'recovery' between each. If you try a number of possible remedies at the same time, you will never know which one is giving the desired effect.

Box 7.	Research in brief: systematic review.

There is a special type of research which can be carried out, known as a 'systematic review'. In this method the researchers scrutinise the results of most of the well-conducted studies into a particular issue, and add these results together to see what evolves. It's very much the principle of 'strength in numbers'. Vogler, Pittler and Ernst (1998) looked at the most rigorous studies into the effectiveness of feverfew in the prevention of migraine. When we are talking about such things as drug trials, 'rigorous' has a particular meaning. It applies to studies called randomised-controlled trials, where one group does get the drug but another, a 'control' group, does not, and the people in both groups are randomly chosen. In Vogler et al.'s research, five studies were identified that had been carried out in such a way. What the researchers found, when looking at the overall results, was that generally feverfew did seem to reduce migraine symptoms in those people taking it. The number of attacks people experienced was lowered, as was the strength of their pain. In addition, people taking feverfew also found themselves vomiting less and generally feeling less nausea. Remember that in the studies included in this research, one group of people was not actually given feverfew, but were given a placebo. A placebo is a substance that cannot have any effects on the body. It is used to fool people into thinking that they are being treated. It allows us to filter out any psychological effects from the effects of the drugs under test. Therefore, in these studies the patients did not know whether they were getting the real drug or the placebo. In the case of feverfew versus placebo, it seems that, generally, the feverfew is effective. This is important, since it seems to counteract the claim that its benefits might only be psychological – that is, the supposition that it only works because you believe in it. If that was the case, the placebo groups would have shown the same effects as the feverfew groups.

Reflexology

Essentially, reflexology is massage of the feet, and occasionally the hands. However, reflexology is based upon a belief that the feet reflect the health of the body generally. Reflexologists work with a 'map' of the feet which shows the areas of the foot that correspond to the areas of the body. There are said to be pathways connecting the foot to the rest of the body, and toxic chemicals can build up in the feet which are harmful to health and show that there is a malfunction elsewhere. Massage of the appropriate areas can break down the crystals (it is claimed), leading to better health. Of course, this may or may not have some truth in it. It largely does not matter. No doctor would argue that a foot massage is not good for you, and will help to relieve stress and therefore pain. Indeed some people who are very sceptical about complementary medicine pay for reflexology because they find it a pleasant and relaxing experience. That alone can be enough. Again, 'emergency' reflexology can avert a headache, and it is possible to massage one's own feet or have a friend or partner do it. While you may lack the skills of someone who has done this thousands of times, you may have some effect, and will not do any harm. It is unlikely to make a headache worse. Even if you are at work, it may be possible to massage your feet, depending upon your type of work or when you can take a break.

Psychological approaches

Psychologists can contribute in a number of ways to the health of those people who experience headaches. Put simply, one of the main inputs of psychology into headache and migraine is where a patient has not been helped by painkillers and the usual medical techniques. Sometimes the only way for a person to deal with pain is psychologically. By helping a person to reassess his or her pain, psychologists can alter the way the pain is experienced. Pain, naturally, creates worry, and worry leads to an enhanced perception of pain. Thus a vicious cycle is established, which a psychologist can help a person to break.

Pain redefinition

One of the ways in which psychologists help with pain involves something called 'pain redefinition'. Put simply, it involves the client developing a different attitude towards the pain. Some people have particularly low pain tolerances and will react very badly to the slightest cut or bump. Such people are the most likely to benefit, in theory, from pain redefinition. By working with a psychologist, they can learn to have less extreme reaction to pain, and, perhaps more crucially, to have more measured and calm thoughts about pain. Instead of panicking, they learn to take pain in their stride and accept it as a part of their life.

Pain redefinition is just a part of something called cognitive-behavioural therapy (CBT) which involves your changing your thoughts, ideas and behaviours. In many cases, CBT can help to reduce your headaches, not directly, but through changes to your lifestyle and your attitude to it. Your doctor can refer you to the psychological services department at your local hospital and, depending upon your problem, you could be seen by any of the specialists there. If you need some kind of lifestyle change you might be helped by a clinical psychologist or a health psychologist.

Sometimes the psychologist can identify other reasons for the persistence of your headaches. If your headaches are due to anxiety and stress as a result of problems in your life, then a counselling psychologist may also be able to help. We all have problems, and there is nothing shameful about admitting it. Men sometimes have particular difficulty admitting to problems, as they often want to convey the impression that they are unshakeable rocks. Well, no one is a rock. It can take a lot of courage to accept that you are fallible, and that you have problems that need help from someone else. If you suspect that your headaches are caused by something that is on your mind, you really should try talking it through with someone, especially someone who is professionally qualified to listen and help you to come to terms with your problems. Some people worry about what counselling involves. It really is nothing unusual. You sit down, confidentially, with someone, and slowly, when you are ready, you talk about your problems. You will not be pushed to talk about anything you do not want to talk about, but the counsellor is someone who is trained to make you feel comfortable about discussing your problems freely. Getting things off your chest is not only a great feeling, but is half of the process of finding a solution. By talking about things that bother you, you will eventually learn to see them in new ways, or perhaps put them more into perspective – and this is almost always a very good thing. This might seem a million miles away from your headaches, but dealing with one set of problems can often help to deal with another. The mind and the body are not separate things. Together they make up the person, and it is the whole person who gets a headache or migraine, not just part of the person.

Relaxation therapy

There is nothing magical or mystical about this, although getting someone to learn to relax is not easy, which is why some people make an occupation of helping others to do so. Have you ever wanted to relax but couldn't? It's not an easy thing to do if you are tense; in fact, some people say that the only time they ever feel really relaxed is when they are asleep. If you can find the time, there are things you can do to relax yourself, but sometimes outside help is also necessary. There is some research to show that regular relaxation does help to combat all sorts of illnesses and all sorts of aches and pains, including migraine and other headaches. If you have tension-type headaches, there is a good chance that proper relaxation is going to make a big difference to your headaches, because stress and lack of relaxation could be the main cause of your headaches in the first place.

If you want to try relaxing by yourself, your local bookshop will stock many appropriate books, but you can also try a few simple things at home. Trying to relax will do you no harm; the worst that can happen is that you will simply not succeed! Be warned, however, that if you do succeed you might find that you doze off to sleep once you are successfully relaxed!

Make sure that you are sitting somewhere very quiet and very comfortable. If you want to play some soft music then this may help. (Many relaxation CDs are commercially available containing the sounds of nature.) Close your eyes, and concentrate on your breathing. Take slow deep breaths. Imagine you are somewhere placid that you would love to be. For many people, this might be on a beach or fishing by the side of a very peaceful river. Imagine the sounds of birds or water around you. Keep concentrating on your breathing. If you think about something stressful instead, like work, then concentrate harder on the nice images such as the sounds of nature around you. Perhaps you can see clouds moving across the sky very slowly or the waves gradually encroaching onto a sandy beach? Do this for 10 or 15 minutes each day. It isn't a long time, but it all adds up. If you can learn to relax in this way, it can have some benefits for both your physical and psychological health.

Hypnosis

Hypnosis, essentially, involves a special kind of relaxation. The hypnotherapist helps you to go into an altered state of consciousness. When you are hypnotised, you may not remember what has happened, so you must trust your hypnotherapist. Most people can be hypnotised, but it only really works on those people who want to be hypnotised. It is a serious business, so don't mistake it for the stage-show hypnotism that you might see on television. In the case of headaches and migraines, hypnotherapy is most likely to be used when a person has headaches of no identifiable origin. If your headaches cannot be attributed to a cause, there is a good chance that they are due to something like stress or anxiety. In these cases, where the cause is psychological, a psychological cure is most likely to be effective. A typical session involves your relaxing in a chair while you are encouraged to fall into a kind of sleep where you can still hear the therapist talking to you and are able to respond. The therapist will help you to defeat your headaches by giving you some coping strategies that work below the level of consciousness. A word of caution: be wary of advertisements that can claim to cure your problem in just one session of hypnotherapy. Try to get your doctor to suggest a good hypnotherapist, or you can find one through the British Psychological Society (BPS). A Chartered Psychologist who practises hypnotherapy is obliged to follow the Code of Conduct of the BPS. There are professional limits on their behaviour, and only a person with sound high-level qualifications in psychology can become a Chartered Psychologist.

Box 8. **Research in brief: the value of hypnosis.**

This piece of research looked at the value of hypnosis in reducing migraine. Emmerson and Trexler (1999) investigated the usefulness of group hypnosis (where a whole group of patients are hypnotised at the same time) and hypnotic relaxation on the severity, duration and frequency of migraines, along with the need for medication. They studied 25 volunteers with migraines who were originally followed for 12 weeks before the hypnosis to check the severity of their normal migraines. After hypnosis, they tracked the subjects' symptoms. Not only did the hypnosis reduce the pain and regularity of the migraines in those taking part, but it also reduced by almost a half the amount of medication that was taken. The average person in the study had a migraine for 54 hours before the hypnosis, and this was brought down to 26 hours. In addition, instead of 3.8 migraine episodes every two weeks, the volunteers were experiencing 2.8. If we work this out per year by multiplying, we can see that hypnosis has made quite a difference to migraineurs. Normally, they were each experiencing an average of 5335 hours annually of migraines. That is a lot of time, especially when you consider that this was reduced to around 1893 hours per year (a reduction of 3442 hours per year, or 57 whole days of pain). Of course, the patients in the study were not subjected to a 12-month follow-up, so we cannot be sure that the benefits of the hypnosis had a continuing effect. However, we at least know that the treatment has the potential to be quite effective.

Combination therapies

In many ways, it is common sense that a combination of medical, complementary and psychological treatments is likely to yield the best results. After all, the cluster of therapies is likely to help to heal both the body and the mind, and neither should be overlooked. Your starting point should be your doctor. Sometimes this is all that is needed. Even with the most horrible migraines, some people can be 'cured' quite easily, even though this is rare. As your doctor works with you to discover the reasons for your headaches, it may then become necessary for you to seek help from complementary sources, and to see a psychologist of some type. The more complicated your headaches, the greater the likelihood that you will need a good combination of therapies. Do not forget, however, that things like social support can be just as important. If you are lucky enough to have friends and family to care for you and help you, then make use of that. If this is a problem, consider joining a support group in your area, or a national society, whether it be for migraine, cluster headaches, menstrual headaches or something else. You should not underestimate the amount of help and information you can receive from such groups. Knowing that you are not alone makes a lot of people feel much better very quickly.

A word on placebo effects

A placebo is a substance or therapy that does not have any physical effect on the functioning of the body but, through psychological means, can alleviate the signs and symptoms of illness and disease. In many books you will find placebo effects considered among complementary therapies, for two reasons. First, some such therapies really seem too far-fetched to be genuinely therapeutic, and indeed are money-making schemes for their practitioners. However, some doctors also have very negative attitudes to complementary therapies. There is an increasing body of research to show that this may be unfair, and that some therapies can have a very real effect some of the time.

However, all medicine – orthodox, psychological or complementary – can be associated with a placebo effect. Essentially, having someone to look after you or take an interest in you makes you feel better. For a host of reasons, this can mean that seeing the doctor is just as likely to have a placebo effect attached to it as seeing a reflexologist or a herbal medicine specialist. However, the amount of placebo effect is what is important. Some therapies seem to be *entirely* a placebo, whereas seeing your doctor rarely is. The drugs and treatments given to you by your doctor are very likely to have a significant effect on your body.

Points to note

- By all means try out complementary therapies, but only when you have already seen your doctor about your headaches.
- Check out your chosen therapy carefully. Not all complementary practitioners are professional and genuine, and many are unregulated.
- Sometimes, psychological help can make a big difference to the quality of your life. Don't be ashamed, worried or afraid about seeking help from the right people.

Where can I get help and information?

One good thing about headaches and migraine is that they are so common that there is a wealth of information and support available. The list below is not comprehensive, and by investigating some of these you will find a 'snowball' effect, with more and more information and advice coming your way. Advice is always variable in quality and in quantity. Not everything you find will be 100 per cent trustworthy, and it is often impossible to police or validate the information you might have access to. The internet presents such a problem. While it can be a valuable source of good-quality, up-to-date information, it also can be the best place to find 'quacks' trying to sell you a fake cure (which in some cases can even make the problem worse) and scaremongers who will frighten you with headache horror stories. By all means use the internet to seek advice, but try to be choosy about which sites you take advice from. Look for some indication that medically qualified personnel are involved, such as by visiting sites run by university medical schools. Avoid sites clearly intended to sell you something, or at least always remember that this is primarily the reason for their existence. If in doubt, be sceptical.

Specialist organisations

The Migraine Action Association, Unit 6, Oakley Hay Lodge Business Park, Great Folds Road, Great Oakley, Northants NN18 9AS. The Migraine Action Association (formerly known as The British Migraine Association) is a charity which, among other things, provides information, publishing leaflets that are distributed to doctors, clinics, libraries and so on. You can visit their website at www.migraine.org.uk.

The Migraine Trust offers information in the form of factsheets, and advice can be found on their website at www.migrainetrust.org.

Books

The Migraine Handbook, by Jenny Lewis, London: Vermilion. A readable and thorough lay guide to migraines endorsed by The Migraine Action Association.

A good starting point for any keen reader of the vast amount of literature available on migraine.

Migraine: Revised and Expanded, by Oliver Sacks, London: Picador. A more academically-oriented book, although still intended for the general reader. This book would probably appeal most to those people who like popular science books. Sacks is a famous neurologist who may be known to you as the author of *Awakenings*, of which a popular film was made. *Migraine* is a wide-ranging book, but tends more towards research and theory into migraines, rather than concentrating on the self-help dimension.

The Complete Idiot's Guide to Migraines and Other Headaches, by Dennis Fox and Jeanne Rejaunier, Indianapolis: Alpha Books. A great bedtime read, with lots of information on just about everything you might want to know about headaches and migraines. Some readers may not like the light-hearted presentation, but others may find it highly readable as a consequence of that.

Migraine for Dummies, by Diane Stafford and Jennifer Shoquist, Chichester: Wiley. Another relatively light-hearted book which covers, in a readable way, the causes and treatments of migraine.

Migraine in Women, by Anne MacGregor, London: Martin Dunitz. A book that outlines the causes of migraines in women and gives tips for management of the migraines associated with pregnancy, menstruation, contraception and HRT.

Medical professionals

In the first instance, your general practitioner is likely to be the best source of advice, especially as to whether your headaches require special treatment or to put your mind at rest that there is nothing to worry about. Depending upon the nature of your headaches, you might be referred to a specialist (consultant). A number of hospitals have specialist headache clinics for this very purpose. You can find a list of these clinics at the Migraine Action Association website; however, you would need a referral letter from your doctor before arranging an appointment with one of these clinics. If you are in the United Kingdom and wish to bypass the National Health Service and pay for specialist advice, there are also a number of private clinics.

Some general practitioners are more than happy to refer people with headaches to consultants, but others are less so. A host of factors may influence this decision, and it is not appropriate to discuss them here. However, if you are in doubt about your doctor's recommendation and believe that you are being 'fobbed off', then you should persevere in trying to seek more help from the medical profession. Please remember to do this nicely, however. Your doctor is much more likely to react favourably to you if you appear to be concerned rather than awkward or petulant. Think how you would react to these statements if you were a doctor:

- I'm still very worried. Is there someone else who could see me just to put my mind at rest? Just in case. . .
- I'm not happy. I think you've got it wrong. I want a second opinion.

The first approach is the best. Doctors are human beings and can be offended or hurt just like anyone. If you treat them respectfully, even if you think they might have made a mistake, you are much more likely to be treated with respect in return.

If you do see a specialist, then he or she is quite likely to be a neurologist. Neurologists look at neurons (nerves), and since the brain is one big collection of nerve cells and pain signals are carried along nerves, neurologists are well placed to study headaches.

Complementary practitioners

The world of complementary therapy is vast and not all practitioners are trustworthy and fair. Some therapies can even be dangerous, and you are advised to tell your doctor of any complementary approaches you are exploring and to research them thoroughly.

In this section, it is only possible to give a small selection of the therapies you might try. Inclusion in this section does not constitute an endorsement, nor does exclusion constitute a warning. The therapies listed here are given because they are relatively common, easy to access, and have shown to have some benefit for some headache and migraine sufferers. Always remember: complementary therapies go alongside orthodox medicine, so **please do not seek complementary medicine *instead* of seeing your doctor**.

Aromatherapy: There are many aromatherapy associations. One of them is The International Federation of Aromatherapists, 182 Chiswick High Road, London W4 1PP.

www.ifaroma.org

Reflexology: The British Reflexology Association, Administration Office, Monks Orchard, Whitbourne, Worcester, WR6 5RB.

www.britreflex.co.uk

Homeopathy: The Society of Homeopaths, 4a Artizan Road, Northampton NN1 4HU.

www.homeopathy-soh.org

Herbalism: National Institute of Medical Herbalists, 56 Longbrook Street, Exeter EX4 6 AH, UK.

www.nimh.org.uk

Chinese Medicine: The British Acupuncture Council, 63 Jeddo Road, London, W12 9HQ.

www.acupuncture.org.uk

The Register of Chinese Herbal Medicine.

www.rchm.co.uk

Therapeutic Massage: Massage Therapy UK offers a long list of practitioners and organisations.

www.massagetherapy.co.uk

The internet

The World Headache Alliance is an international alliance of headache-related organisations. The website is excellent and features details of research articles, tips on relieving headaches, and headache news. It includes a section on medical and psychological evidence-based research into headaches. If you liked the Research in Brief sections in this book, you might want to investigate this site for more detailed information.

www.w-h-a.org/

The International Headache Society, allied to the World Headache Alliance, is a professional, medical society devoted to the research of, and debate about, headaches. Some of the information on the site is patient-friendly.

www.i-h-s.org/

Clusterheadaches.com is a world-wide support group and discussion forum for people with cluster headaches. It is a well-maintained and interesting site.

www.clusterheadaches.com

The Organisation for the Understanding of Cluster Headache have a website that should be accessed for British-based information and advice.

www.ouch-uk.org.

Headachecare.com is a site maintained by a network of primary care providers (general practitioners). It has some interesting information, including a quick diagnostic quiz (with which the usual caution must be taken).

www.headachecare.com/

MIDAS have a questionnaire that can help to identify the extent to which your migraine disables you in life. The Migraine Disability Assessment Questionnaire is downloadable in a variety of languages from the website.

www.midas-migraine.net

The Migraine Awareness Group provides information at

www.migraines.org.

The British Association for the Study of Headache is an academic and professional association. If you have an appropriate academic or clinical background then this organisation will be of interest to you, but less so if you are a migraine patient.

www.bash.org.uk

Points to note

- Your local library should be able to give you a lot of information on headaches and migraine.
- Use the internet carefully, perhaps sticking only to the sites recommended in this book.

- Do not scare yourself by reading lots of medical textbooks. The vast majority of headaches are *not* life threatening or serious, even though they can be painful and alarming.
- Do not be afraid to seek help from your doctor. He or she is a very good source of help and information.

Checklist

This list is intended to help you to determine the type of headache you are likely to be experiencing. It has been checked and agreed by a doctor who specialises in headaches and migraines; however, it is not intended to replace a doctor's diagnosis, which you are strongly advised to seek as a matter of course. Remember that if a headache is unusually severe, or has lasted a long time (more than a day or two), or is the result of an injury such as a blow to the head, see a doctor immediately. Do not forget that if your headache is very strong, or you are dizzy or very sensitive to light, **do not drive**. Find some other way to see the doctor. Get a friend or partner to take you, or even ask your doctor to call.

The checklist works on a majority basis. Work through all of the sections, ticking boxes where the statement applies to you. When done, look back over the whole list. You ought to have ticked more boxes in one section than in any other. If that is true, then you probably have the headache type listed in that category. If you have a equal number of ticks in two categories, then it is possible that you actually do have more than one kind of headache affecting you. This is exactly why you need to speak with your doctor.

Tension-type headache

It feels like there is a tight band around my head. ☐
My neck or shoulders hurt, and my neck is stiff when I move. ☐
If I feel around, I can often find a sore spot on the side of my head, near ☐
   the temple.
The headache is constant. ☐
The headache can get worse if I bend down or push on the toilet. ☐
My temperature is normal. ☐

Chronic headache

You will probably experience the symptoms listed under tension-type headaches, but:

I have headaches which can last a few days. ☐
My headaches have been going on for at least six months. ☐
I have as many as 15 days of headache every month. ☐

Migraine without aura

The pain is on one side of my head. ☐
The pain is throbbing. ☐
I am hypersensitive to light. ☐
I am hypersensitive to sound. ☐
I cannot find the words to talk. ☐
I need to find a quiet dark place and sleep. ☐
I feel sick or actually vomit. ☐
My temperature is normal. ☐
The pain can last up to 72 hours. ☐
Physical activity can make things worse. ☐

Migraine with aura

This is the same as migraine without aura, but in addition you might experience some other signs or symptoms.

Before my headaches start, I experience one or more of these:

dizziness ☐
numbness ☐
pins and needles ☐
an odd taste or smell ☐
a curve of light spreading across my view ☐
flashing lights ☐

Cluster headache

The pain is absolutely excruciating. ☐
The pain is sharp or stabbing. ☐
The pain is mainly in my eye socket area. ☐

My eye or nose streams. ☐

My eyelid droops. ☐

My pupil in the eye on the affected side is smaller than the other. ☐

I sometimes find myself walking around or 'dancing' to cope ☐
with the pain.

My temperature is normal. ☐

The attacks occur in clusters of up to eight a day for a few weeks or ☐
months.

The pain usually lasts no more than a couple of hours. ☐

Other headaches and symptoms

If you are about to tick any of these boxes, please see a doctor as soon as possible as you might have a condition that requires immediate treatment.

The pain is sudden and very strong. ☐

I have experienced numbness on one side of the body. ☐

I have been vomiting AND have a high temperature. ☐

I felt like someone hit me with a baseball bat on the back of the neck. ☐

References and further reading

These are the full references for the articles mentioned in the *Research in Brief* boxes of this book. Unless you have an academic/medical background they are *not* recommended as a source of information. They can be quite technical, and understanding their research findings usually involves some understanding of quite advanced statistical procedures.

Emmerson, G.J. & Trexler, G. (1999). An hypnotic intervention for migraine control. *Australian Journal of Clinical and Experimental Hypnosis, 27,* 54–61.

Holm, J.E., Bury, L. & Suda, K.T. (1996). The relationship between stress, headache and the menstrual cycle in young female migraineurs. *Headache, 36,* 531–537.

MacGregor, E.A. (1997). The doctor and the migraine patient: improving compliance. *Neurology, 48* (Supplement 3), S16–S20.

Marlowe, N. (1998). Self-efficacy moderates the impact of stressful events on headache. *Headache, 38,* 662–667.

Meyer, J.S., Thornby, J., Crawford, K. & Rauch, G.M. (2000). Reversible cognitive decline accompanies migraine and cluster headaches. *Headache, 40,* 638–646.

Torelli, P., Cologno, D. & Manzoni, G.C. (1999). Weekend headache: a possible role of work and life-style. *Headache, 39,* 398–408.

Vogler, B.K., Pittler, M.H. & Ernst, E. (1998). Feverfew as a preventive treatment for migraine: a systematic review. *Cephalalgia, 18,* 704–708.

Further reading

If you wish to read more about headaches and migraine, the following books are recommended. There are many others, but these are some of the author's favourites.

Fox, D. & Rejaunier, J. (2000). *The Complete Idiot's Guide to Migraines and Other Headaches.* Indianapolis: Alpha.

Lewis, J. (1998). *The Migraine Handbook: The definitive guide to the causes, symptoms and treatments.* London: Vermilion.

Lockley, J. (1993). *Headaches: A comprehensive guide to relieving headaches and migraine*. London: Bloomsbury.

Sacks, O. (1995). *Migraine. Revised and expanded edition*. London: Picador.

Stafford, D. & Shoquist, J. (2003). *Migraines for Dummies*. Chichester: John Wiley & Sons.

Trickett, S. (1999). *Coping with Headaches*. London: Sheldon Press.

Index

What is visual stress? Why do coloured overlays work?

"Optometrists and pediatricians will also find this work to be a valuable resource. It is a 'must read'"

Alan Kwasman M.D., *Behavioural Pediatrician*

0-470-85116-3
March 2003
£15.99
€24.00
Paperback

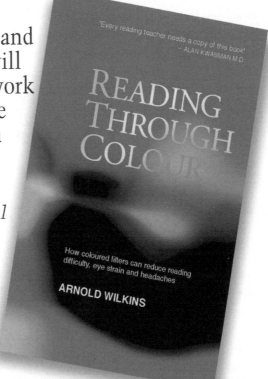

'Every reading teacher needs a copy of this book'
— ALAN KWASMAN M.D

READING THROUGH COLOUR

How coloured filters can reduce reading difficulty, eye strain and headaches

ARNOLD WILKINS

Order your copy today!
visit www.wileyeurope.com

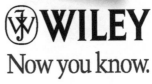

WILEY
Now you know.

wileyeurope.com

All prices correct at time of going to press, but subject to change.

5275

The 'Understanding Illness and Health' series

New titles for 2004!

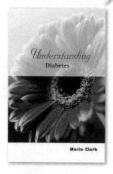

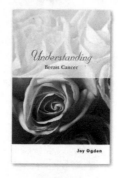

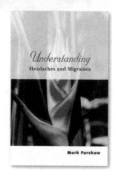

Understanding Diabetes
0-470-85034-5 • Paper
January 2004 • £9.99

Understanding Breast Cancer
0-470-85435-9 • Paper
March 2004 • £9.99

Understanding Headaches
0-470-84760-3 • Paper
February 2004 • £9.99

Also available in this series...

Understanding Childhood Eczema
0-470-84759-X
Paper
2003

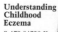

Understanding Irritable Bowel Syndrome
0-470-84496-5
Paper
2003

Understanding Menopause
0-470-84471-X
Paper
2003

Understanding Skin Problems
0-470-84518-X
Paper
2003

All books can be purchased at good bookshops or online at www.wileyeurope.com

All prices are correct at time of going to press but subject to change

WILEY

Now you know.

wileyeurope.com

Clear, balanced, positive advice....to help you cope.

5342